MYTHIN
EXCUSE

Understanding, Recognizing, and Overcoming Eating Disorders

LISA MESSINGER
MERLE CANTOR GOLDBERG, LCSW

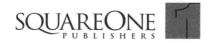

SQUAREONE
PUBLISHERS

The information and advice contained in this book are based upon the research and the personal and professional experiences of the author. They are not intended as a substitute for consulting with a health care professional. The publisher and author are not responsible for any adverse effects or consequences resulting from the use of any of the suggestions, preparations, or procedures discussed in this book. All matters pertaining to your physical health should be supervised by a health care professional. It is a sign of wisdom, not cowardice, to seek a second or third opinion.

Since this book is based on her real life, Lisa Messinger has changed the character names, physical descriptions, and other details regarding people's lives. Ms. Goldberg has done the same regarding any case histories she mentions.

A Note on Gender: To avoid long and awkward phrasing within sentences, the female pronouns are used when referring to a person with an eating disorder. This is not meant to suggest that males do not suffer from eating disorders, as eating disorders affect both men and women.

Square One Publishers

115 Herricks Road
Garden City Park, NY 11040
(516) 535-2010 • (877) 900-BOOK
www.squareonepublishers.com

COVER DESIGNER: Jeannie Tudor
EDITOR: Elaine Weiser
TYPESETTER: Gary A. Rosenberg

Library of Congress Cataloging-in-Publication Data

Messinger, Lisa
    My thin excuse : understanding, recognizing, and overcoming eating
disorders / Lisa Messinger and Merle Cantor Goldberg.
        p. cm.
    Includes index.
    ISBN-13: 978-0-7570-0259-5 (pbk.)
    ISBN-10: 0-7570-0259-5 (pbk.)
    1. Eating disorders—Popular works. I. Cantor Goldberg, Merle. II. Title.

RC552.E18M47   2006
616.85'26—dc22

2006023581

Printed in Canada

10   9   8   7   6   5   4   3   2   1

Contents

This book is dedicated to my husband, Joel,
who has been an ear, a shoulder, a huge heart, and,
fortunately, the whole incredible loving package
inside and out through thick and thin.

—L.M.

To my loving husband, Walter Goozh,
and my unique and very special daughter, Stephanie Goozh.
I love you both very much.

To Col. Stanley L. Cantor and Alberta Gottfried Cantor,
my parents, who taught me,
by their incomparable example, how to live.

—M.G.

Acknowledgments

Thanks to all the talented people at Square One, especially publisher Rudy Shur, who has been a wonderful friend and mentor to me for many years; editor Elaine Weiser, whose work is so helpful, thorough, and thoughtful; and publicity and marketing director Anthony Pomes, who is always brimming with good ideas. Warm remembrances of the late John Arena, a caring soul everyone should be lucky enough to have as their first publisher, who paid such special attention to me and this subject matter. Thanks and love to my mother, who is always there no matter what, no matter when; my father, for caring enough to learn to understand; and my brother, a great friend as well as relative.

—L.M.

First and foremost I wish to thank Rudy Shur and Anthony Pomes for their invaluable guidance, continuing insights, and learning. To Elaine Weiser, a model of editing expertise, patience, and empathetic understanding. To my colleagues at IAEDP, through so many years of teaching and learning together—always reaching for the gold standard. To Dr. Marie Shafe, a brilliant and dedicated educator and true friend. To Caroline Miller, coach, author, and role model, and to Janet Greeson, dedicated professional who introduced me to the field so many years ago. To the late Dr. Carl Goldberg, a brilliant and prolific writer, clinician, and mentor, always encouraging me to write and unselfishly sharing concepts and ideas. To my wonderful family—Walter and Stephanie Goozh; Diane, Julian, and Justin Astley; Cynthia and Chris Brown; Jennifer Bergman; Wendy, Jerry, Eric, Jen, Brady, and Craig Santoro; Joanne and Nate Sternberg; and mom-mom. I promise to come out of my study now (at least for a while).

And finally to Lisa, with respect and admiration.

—M.G.

Introduction

There always used to be a few candy wrappers under my bed. Not candy *bar* wrappers, but candy *bag* wrappers. I used to eat bags of candy, bags of cookies, bags of junk food, cartons of ice cream, dozens of doughnuts, and entire cakes. I wasn't fat. I wasn't hungry. I wasn't even a food-lover. I had an eating disorder.

I was a bulimic, someone who binges and purges. Actually, in terms of my physical health, I was more fortunate than some bulimics. I didn't vomit. Nevertheless, I fell within the ever-widening recognized spectrum of people with serious eating disorders, those with unreasonable, life-consuming concerns regarding body, weight, and eating. This huge and quickly growing group includes everyone from rail-thin anorectics to those plump from compulsive overeating. If you are holding this book, you or someone you love is probably a member of this very nonexclusive, yet extremely scary, and often life-threatening, club. My form of purging was not vomiting, but it was a "purge," a way to "purify" myself. It was a way to rid myself not only of calories, but of the guilt I felt over eating. Like millions of others, I was caught in an addictive cycle of binging, followed by starvation dieting and compulsive exercise—not occasionally, but every day. Like all of us with any of the varied eating disorders along the spectrum, I was a slave to a scale and a twisted set of self-imposed rules.

It's hard to remember those rules. I did, however, write most of them down in my diary. The front cover read "One Year Diary," next to which I wrote, "You wanna make a bet!" That's because I wrote sporadically in that diary for over seven years, from the ages of fifteen through twenty-two. It tells my story and I have a feeling it tells yours, too, or one like it. Because we who are entangled in self-destructive, energy-consuming cycles are far from alone.

This book came about because Francine Snyder, my psychologist who specialized in eating disorders, asked if she could include some of my writing in a project she was putting together. There was my diary, a few journals, a lot of assorted papers, and a couple of scrapbooks. A number of my writing instructors at the University of Southern California, where I was a journalism major, encouraged journal writing as class exercises. After seeing my entries, they also strongly suggested I have my diary published. As I read over my diary, journals, and papers, I realized that, without trying, I had caught on paper the obsession and compulsion of an eating disorder. I had written about it almost at its birth, before I even knew what it was, right through my recovery. I knew immediately my diary and journals, which intimately revealed everything about my life, including my rituals, secrets, and eventual therapeutic break-throughs, could help others like you.

People living with an eating disorder are often secretive and find few out-lets for their real feelings. Writing for me was partly this, but it was also more. I always wanted to be a writer. And I always wrote even when I didn't know I wanted to be a writer. While I was in college, I had my first professional sub-mission accepted by a national magazine. The editor of the magazine then asked me, a nineteen year old, to be a contributing reporter. I went on to get my degree in journalism, with a minor in women's studies, and have gone on to be a nationally award-winning health, nutrition, and food journalist, syndi-cated columnist, and the author or coauthor of seven books.

I say this in order to provide some perspective on why I thought my diary might speak to you. I may have been suffering with the trauma of an eating disorder through the years this book covers; however, I was always a writer. The book that follows was never merely "Dear Diary." Although I never expected anyone else to read it, I was always, for some reason, addressing my thoughts "Dear World."

As it developed, however, this work blossomed into much more than a diary, and that is why I know it will be of even more help to you or your loved one. Through my work as a health, medical, and nutrition journalist, editor, and book author, I was fortunate to be recommended to work as editorial consultant for Merle Cantor Goldberg, LCSW, BCD, on another book. Merle is one of the country's leading eating-disorders psychotherapists and a longtime leader of the International Association of Eating Disorders Professionals Insti-tute. I knew her cutting-edge, therapeutic perspective could analyze my diary and add possibly lifesaving advice for you.

Therefore, each time you read a few compelling, emotional chapters of the diary, you will then get helpful information (we call them *Insights*) from Merle. You will undoubtedly find highly relatable the diary's *What's Wrong With Me?* and *I'll Diet 'Til I Drop* chapters, as I struggle with discovering and understanding my "strange eating habits" and start monitoring every morsel that goes into my mouth amidst the backdrop of being a "perfect" straight-A student, varsity tennis player, and award-winning public speaker. I was also a friend, girlfriend, sister, and daughter, but never told anyone close to me—except my diary—about my struggle with food. Merle brings a brilliant focus on everything I write about early in the diary in her immensely helpful chap-ter, *How to Identify an Eating Disorder*, which includes the most comprehensive explanations of the entire spectrum of eating disorders that I have ever seen.

In *Itsy-Bitsy-Teeny-Weeny Polka-Dot Bikini,* I achieve the ultimate dream of all of us with eating disorders. Although I was never fat, except in my own mind, I finally starve and exercise myself into becoming exceptionally thin and what I—and the even more men with whom I am coming into contact, including tall blond models at my new coveted job on the sets of America's top television shows—consider to be the "perfect" woman. A euphoria that you, too, at times may have experienced, sets in here. It all quickly falls apart, though, in *Overwhelmed,* where I almost break down trying to understand why that perfection and weight loss is not providing lasting happiness. Merle's *Getting Thin Is Not the Answer* tells us all why our ultimate goal of thinness, even when met, will just lead to additional problems if we don't determine our underlying motivations.

In *Limbo, White-Knuckling It,* and *Momentary Hell,* I begin to eat meagerly again rather than completely starve myself, and desperately try to go it alone and tick off the seemingly interminable days one-by-one that I've been "good." Even with that glamorous TV job and nights filled with exciting dates, I force myself to eat by impossibly strict rules in a frantic attempt to stay thin. If I had read Merle's *Insights* section on page 127 *Why Self-Treatment Doesn't Work* then, I would have understood that my solo attempts would always be futile. I would have saved myself a lot of pain and stress, and I am so grateful that you or someone you care about can reap the benefits of her wisdom.

I finally begin to see Francine Snyder, a psychologist specializing in eating disorders, as well as attend an eating disorders support group at the University of Southern California, and I capture in my diary the breakthroughs the moment I have them. In *Weekly Therapy, Skipping Sessions,* and *Promises, Promises,* I realize for the first time that this daily, self-destructive prison of a vicious cycle literally has nothing to do with food or weight. That amazed me and I am grateful to have caught this vital process on paper so that it can also trigger flashes of recognition from you. Merle's *Seeking Help for Yourself or Someone You Care About* will take you far beyond those flashes to concrete, specific, life-altering advice.

No one said it was going to be easy. *Love Affair* and *Real Life* catch the extreme highs, as well as occasional setbacks, that are part of living life on your own two feet without the harmful crutch of an eating disorder. In my case, that might have included a new sense of true self-confidence, dating and marrying a talented actor (who enters my life in the final diary chapter of this book), and working as a globe-trotting reporter. But it also meant dealing with what I finally realized were the often-extreme stresses of life—including the ups and downs of weight loss and weight gain—rather than numbing them with the compulsion of food binges followed by starvation and excessive exercise.

Merle's *Advice for the Rest of Your Life* further explores all of that and adds invaluable guidance that will help ensure you or someone you love may never get caught again in the dangerous trap of an eating disorder.

If you are concerned that you or someone you care about may have signs of an eating disorder, reading this book will provide valuable information and insight into the disease. Sometimes these signs can be subtle, sometimes not so subtle. The checklist, *Recognizing an Eating Disorder*, can help you identify the presence of a problem in yourself or a loved one. Turn to page 6 for the questionnaire. Then, continue reading to learn more about this life-threatening issue.

Problem? What Problem?

With any eating disorder, early detection is essential so that treatment can begin before the disorder spins completely out of control and before substantial medical damage occurs. The problem is that early on, the eating disorder may be difficult to detect for friends and family, and even if you, yourself, have the eating disorder, you may feel (like Lisa) confused by what is occurring, or in denial about the severity of the changes in yourself that you are seeing. As in Lisa's case, the path may begin slowly and insidiously, and before you know it, take over almost all aspects of your thoughts and actions. If you are concerned about yourself or a loved one, ask yourself the following questions and answer "yes" or "no." It is important to be as honest as possible about your feelings and observations.

The checklist on the next page is designed to help you get more in touch with what is happening to you or someone you love. It is hard to pinpoint an exact number of "yes" responses that would indicate or not indicate an eating disorder. Although some are normal signs of adolescence, all of the "yes" answers are significant and bear further thought. However, more than five "yes" responses to the above questions give additional cause for concern.

If you are reading this list for yourself, some of the questions may make a lot of sense and shed additional light on what you may be experiencing. Do not be afraid to look inside. There is nothing to be embarrassed about or ashamed of and *you are not alone.* If you are reading this list with someone you love in mind, there is also no need to be afraid. Trust your intuition. You probably know this person well, and what you are most looking for is a major change, particularly in terms of weight and food, from the person's normal behavior.

If you answer "yes" to five or more of the following questions, you may be suffering from an eating disorder. It is important to seek help, and remember that there are people out there who can offer real help. However, my telling you to seek help may not do the trick. The trick is in recognizing the signs yourself and taking back control of your life!

Recognizing an Eating Disorder

Circle your responses to the following questions.
After tallying your answers, turn to page 5 for more information.

In terms of food behaviors:

1. Has there been any radical change or sudden shift
    in food behaviors—anything about your eating that
    is very different from before?   **Yes   No**

2. Is there an increasing preoccupation with food,
    "healthy eating," vegetarianism, diet, fat content?
    Are you reading recipes more and thinking about the
    next meal much of the time?   **Yes   No**

3. Is there an unexplained change in eating habits?
    Are you creating rules around food and eating?   **Yes   No**

4. Are you skipping meals with family or friends, very picky
    about food, or severely limiting portions as you move
    your food around your plate to avoid detection? Do
    you say or feel you are not hungry a lot or feel bloated
    or fat when eating normal amounts of food? Are you
    losing touch with your hunger and fullness cues?   **Yes   No**

5. Are you eating excessive amounts of food usually
    alone and in a hidden place? Does this make you
    feel out of control, ashamed, or guilty?   **Yes   No**

6. Do you label foods "good" or "bad"? Do you label
    yourself "good" or "bad" in terms of your food
    intake for the day?   **Yes   No**

7. Are you drinking large amounts of non-caloric, diet
    soda, water, or iced tea?   **Yes   No**

8. Are you leaving the table immediately after meals to go
    to the rest room? Has there been a radical change in
    weight with frequent "weigh-ins" several times a day?
    Do you avoid being weighed by anyone else or letting
    anyone else see your weight?   **Yes   No**

9. Are you wearing baggy clothes to hide your weight loss/
gain? Do you avoid situations, like shopping or beaches,
where others might see you in revealing or little clothes?   **Yes   No**

10. Have you begun to define yourself by your food?
Your weight? Your exercise routine?   **Yes   No**

In terms of health:

11. Do you put on extra layers of clothing to keep warm?
Are you frequently cold?   **Yes   No**

12. Have you been missing your menstrual cycle?   **Yes   No**

13. Is your skin dry or flaky, your hair very dull, dry or
brittle, and/or nails breaking?   **Yes   No**

14. Are you experiencing tooth pain and decay much
more often than before?   **Yes   No**

In terms of moods and behavior:

15. Do your moods seem up and down lately in a way
that is very different from what you are used to?
Are they sometimes difficult to control?   **Yes   No**

16. Are you very afraid of gaining weight?   **Yes   No**

17. Are you questioning your relationships more?
More overly sensitive?   **Yes   No**

18. Do you want to be alone more lately?   **Yes   No**

19. Do you feel like just not talking as much, not doing
as much as before, or just not as interested in what
you used to be?   **Yes   No**

20. Have you become overly involved with one activity,
such as studying, to a degree that is different or
surprising, or that creates too much anxiety or
tension? Does that activity tend to be isolating?   **Yes   No**

21. Do you feel self-conscious or embarrassed more or
are you much more aware of how you appear to
others?   **Yes   No**

22. Is it harder to just relax and be spontaneous? Is it hard to remain happy? Do you feel like crying without knowing why?   **Yes   No**

23. Is a sense of control much more important than it used to be? Do you feel like you are always struggling to beat the stress around you when it seems almost impossible to do? Do you feel like you are beginning to lose control?   **Yes   No**

24. Are you exercising more than 1–2 hours a day? Are you upset when you are not able to perform your exercise routine? Do you center your day around exercise?   **Yes   No**

Add up your "yes' and "no" answers: **Total**   ____ ____

1. What's Wrong With Me?

15 TO 17 YEARS OLD

"Tomorrow is the first day of the rest of my life!" I'm turning over a new leaf. I will no longer be shy. I will be confident. I will be able to talk with boys with ease. I won't wonder if I look good. I will look good.

The biggest thing on my mind is the math test. I'll try my best. (I hope I do good! Real good!!) I guess I'm afraid of not doing well. I feel like everyone expects so much of me, including me.

I'm going to act the way I used to with Joe, insults and all. I still want him to be my friend. I guess I'm just jealous. I hate hearing boys like Joe talking about other girls. What's wrong with me? They treat me as though I were nothing but a huge brain! I hate being classified as that! Just because I get all A's doesn't mean I'm not a normal girl.

Shelly's "interested look" is driving me crazy! I guess it's bothering me because I was jealous when they said how good at tennis she was.

Today, I have to say, I was really flabbergasted. At lunch, Staci very bluntly informed me that she'd appreciate it if I'd stop spreading rumors about her! Well, I had no idea what she was talking about. She went on muttering that I said that she got a C on a test and that I would have cried if it had been me. I knew what she meant. I had told Cindy something similar (not word for word) to that about two weeks ago. There was nothing wrong with me telling my best friend how I felt about someone! Cindy told Staci something I had told her in private. I felt like crying. I'm going to call Cindy and talk this out. I'm sure, since she was sitting right there, she knows I'm upset with her. Something else bothered me. All my friends (?) just sat there as Staci preached my wrongdoings. It was as if they had already heard the story.

Well, I got a B+ on my world studies test. I think one question away from an A. I was disappointed, but recovered. Got an A on my Spanish test. Hallelujah! I thought I might never see another one. Thought I was slipping. I guess I've finally got my footing again!

Why can't I giggle? Why can't I sit around at lunch and giggle and talk about

West Valley High School
Abuela School District

Office of Principal
The Parent Faculty Club
Music Boosters

Miss Lisa Messinger
7089 Cardinal Drive
Encino, California

Dear Lisa:

Well, you did it again! Another perfect semester! I'm really
impressed with your academic achievement and can assure you, as
a result, you will reap many fine rewards. The really neat part
is that in addition to the perfect grades, you found time to
participate in our speech and debate and tennis programs thus
disproving the "Book Worm Theory."

Maintaining a 4.0 grade point average is not an easy task and
I commend you for your accomplishment. Most people fail to
realize the effort that is necessary to achieve this level of
scholarship. It takes motivation, dedication, and, above all,
hard work. You have apparently set high goals for yourself and
have demonstrated the willingness to give high priority to
them. Your parents must be very proud and pleased with your
success and I am sure they also deserve a pat on the back.

Enclosed you will find your well-earned "Outstanding 'A'
Student Pass."

The future should hold many interesting experiences for you and
I am looking forward to the opportunity of guiding you through
the remainder of your high school years.

    Sincerely,

    Jerry Wise

    Jerry Wise
    Principal

boys? Why do I have to go to the library and study? Why do I feel mortified sitting around with a bunch of giggling girls?

I don't know what to do. If I leave them, these friends from junior high school and even elementary school, I will have no one. But having no one is beginning to seem more and more preferable.

I couldn't believe it when they started cutting Joe down right in front of me. They know what good friends we are. And they're just jealous. Joe's on the baseball team and the honor roll, and what do they have, nothing! Forget it, I think I'll just take Joe and take my chances and just move on. Forget this. We are so different.

JULY 1

Joe is my boyfriend! Jim Michaels called! Richard Gold called last week. Well, I've done it! I'm at ease with boys and not so unpopular either! I guess I'm proud. Joe says he's in love with me. I'm skeptical. We've been joking friends for so long, I couldn't believe it when he kissed me and told me he loved me. I *know* I'm not in love with anyone now! I really do like him, though, and I like kissing, too. That surprises me, but I'm curious to find out what comes next. Although I almost slammed the door in his face when he tried more than the tiniest little kiss. Well, I hope John Stern isn't getting any ideas, because I'm not. Joe. Joe. Joe.

Well, I still hope to grow.

P.S. I've escaped from those idiotic, immature friends, who were not really friends at all.

JULY 2

At first it's just jokes, insults too,
You're sure that he despises you.
Then he calls for an assignment, says everyone else is out.
"You've been on the phone for two hours!" you hear your mother shout.
You never knew you could find so much to talk about.

Back at school, you're closer than ever.
But, as to being more than friends, never.
You can talk about anything and everything.
Why is it you nearly jump every time you hear the phone ring?
You feel close, true, but it lacks that special "zing."

The last day of school is finally here.
In his eyes, could it be a trace of fear?
The yearbooks are signed, and you see you haven't passed the joking stage.

But, still, you search for a hidden message on the page.

The play's over. We were actors, the classroom our stage.

But, wait! He walks you home, there's a kiss, and nothing will ever, can ever, be the same.

AUGUST 1

Well, we just drifted apart. Phooey! I go to Hawaii for two weeks with Mom and Dad and my brother and we never see each other again. That really makes a lot of sense!

Joe is immature. He tells me he loves me, and then I go to Hawaii for my brother's bar mitzvah gift and he never calls again. I can't call him. I used to be able to when it was for homework or something. Not about this.

I don't even care. This was not working out, these two weeks of him telling me that when we're sixteen he'll get away from his family and we'll get married.

I'm not going anywhere when I'm sixteen. Besides, I don't even like kissing him, the little that I did.

There's got to be a lot more to see than this.

NOVEMBER 10

I'm on the verge of a new beginning. I can feel it! Get this, now I'm the one starting the conversations with boys. Mark Jefferson saying how cute I am. It's the first time I may not get A's. I may get a B+ in algebra II (maybe an A-). Me and Joe, we're always continuing. Things were very awkward after our stormy, not to mention short, romance. But *I* broke the ice. I called him on Halloween (for help in math, ha-ha). We're friends like always again. Relief. To be more than friends is just too complicated. He is, though, an extremely special person.

Things are really going well. My sweet sixteen party!!! Rob Jeffries a possible guest. Wow! One boyfriend . . . not for me, today anyway. I'm happy. I'm actually confident. I have a feeling that things will get even better, too. I really felt strongly about Mike. Then, all of a sudden I changed my mind. Well, from now on it's me, me, me. I keep thinking about what was with Joe and me. What does that mean, Doctor?

Terri, Kim (a new friend I really like), Amy. They're a new group. They're smart, they play tennis, they're nice, and they'll do for now. I still want to grow with boys and girls.

The real me is a pretty, smart, attractive and even sexy girl. The me that shows is insecure, aloof, and inferior feeling. Why? And, can I change?

Happiness isn't the word. I don't know what the word is, but I feel good about me! Sixteen years old and I gave a sweet sixteen party (never thought I could). It really did go pretty well. Kim. Finally a friend that seems just right for me. Mike. I can't believe it, I asked him to the Sadie Hawkins' Dance. I just hope it all works out. Nothing really special yet, but I do like him a lot. Joe. Still in the picture, I really care about him. I can't pinpoint the feeling, talk about confusing! Rob. A hope for the future. I'm not that taken with him, even though he's beautiful and gorgeous and smart. I guess that proves something. I'm looking, waiting, for true love. It still seems a long way off.

A's. I got them. It really is important.

I told Joe how I felt about his teasing me all the time. It felt good. Lilli. I have to admit I was jealous. Why? I don't know, way inside.

Lucky I'm never really unhappy. But right now I'm happy not because of one specific thing, just because I'm me.

Dear Lilli,

It's been a while, how are you? I can't stand this weather.

February 24 is the school's first semi-formal Sadie Hawkins' Dance, I got my courage up and asked (guess who?), remember Mike? Well, that's who I asked. He said that he'd love to. I got an outfit yesterday, a light blue dress. I think we might do something before or after.

Lilli, I really wish you were here instead of all the way in Antelope Valley. I know it's only an hour away, but still! So much has been happening, and while my mom tries to understand she's got her own ideas. Make sure nobody reads this. Write back soon. Maybe you can give me some advice.

Remember Joe? Well, he compared us again. He told me I should wear a lower, more suggestive shirt, he said that's what boys like. When he saw I wasn't paying attention, he said, "You're no fun. Your cousin Lilli is fun, she doesn't act disgusted to hear stuff like you, you just act like you hate it."

And then the other day right in math, Joe starts telling me what a "good girl" I am, never did a thing wrong in my life. Then he says he can't wait to see me after I "lose my virginity." He said it'll probably be when I'm 35 and married. Then he said, "Who knows? It might be Mike!" I was getting mad. He said that now that I was 16 I was desperate for sex, and that's why *I* was going after Mike (ha-ha). Then he said he wanted to give me some advice about taking Mike to the dance. I told him to shut up, so he wrote me a note saying that all Mike wants is sex, and that I better give it to him or he won't go. You know, I've been called "sweet" and "saint" and "perfect" a lot these past weeks. If you act like you like a boy, does that mean he'll think you want him to try something?

We had carnations for sale for Valentine's Day. I sent one to Richard Gold, who I really do like and probably should have asked to the Sadie Hawkins' Dance. I also sent one to Rod Burke (his brother told my brother that he's madly in love with me), also to Jim Stern, and, you won't believe it, to Joe (before he gave me his sex education lecture).

I ran my jog-a-thon, 18 laps in an hour. Not that fantastic, but it was fun.

So, what's new in your always exciting life? How's Craig? Is he still going for Heather or has he realized that you're the one for him? Well, I hope you can come and stay over spring break. Please write back soon, especially what you think of all this with Joe and Mike.

Love,
Lisa

FEBRUARY 17

Dear Lilli,

Well, I'm glad you wrote back so fast. How was your Valentine's Day? Discover any secret admirers? The carnations delivered at school turned out to be plants, because the flowers got ruined by rain. They were cute—you wrote a little message and the person got it in their class. I didn't think I'd get any, but I got one from Rod (the cute one who I think is so sweet). He just wrote, "Always, Rod." I kinda wish I asked him to the Sadie Hawkins' Dance, but, anyway, I sent him one too.

I'm really glad that I did ask Mike to the dance. After all, these guys may be cute and on the basketball team, but they're more friends (although I'd go out with them)! But Mike (who is, of course, also on the basketball team!) is the one I've thought and thought and thought about. All this time, I mean way back when Joe proclaimed his love for me, it was Mike—his best friend—who I had the crush on. I've never felt this strongly before. It's like I can't control myself. I think about him all the time. He's so charming and smart and CUTE! I decided I'm not wearing the blue dress to the dance. It's just too much. I'm going to get something else.

Well, I've got another question for my cousin, the authority. If a guy really likes you a lot and you like him as a good friend and that's it, how would you handle it if he wants you to like him like he likes you? Who I'm talking about is Jim Stern, I think I really hurt him. He wants me to go to the basketball party, and I say sure. He wants me to go out with him when he gets his car, and I say sure. He asks me if I've asked someone to the dance, and I say sure. Not sure, but yes. I could tell he thought I really liked him. I don't see anything wrong with liking lots of guys, do you? Why tie yourself down when you can do lots of things with lots of people? Although, all I really want is for Mike to like me.

My mom's ideas . . . I don't know. I just think that some time I might really want to give/get more than a goodnight kiss. Not much more. What are your thoughts on this?

Write back soon and tell me about you and Craig. I hope everything with Gus works out too! I'll certainly have a lot of news next time about the dance!!!!!!

Love,
Lisa

FEBRUARY 20

Well, this is the worst day of my life. Period. I feel awful. I cried all night. Not one hour. Not two hours. All night.

I called my mom at her card game. I've never done that. I just couldn't believe it. I was so upset.

I was baking cookies, and Mike called. He can't go. I bought two outfits, and he can't go. He lied, too. I didn't think so when he called, but now I know.

He said his mom was going out of town and he had to go to his dad's house in Orange County. One day before the dance! I said, "Can't you stay with Ken?" "No," he said, "my mom said, no. I promised my dad."

When I got off the phone I couldn't stop crying, and I called my mom.

Then, yesterday, the *day of the dance*, I couldn't believe it. I got my driver's license, passed the test, was driving with my mom for the first time up my street, and who do I see, Joe and Mike! I said to my mom, "That's Joe and Mike, they're walking up to *our* house. Don't look!"

At home I made my brother look out the window, and there they were! They started walking around in my back yard! I went out and said, "You're trespassing." They said they were just going around and bothering everyone they knew named Lisa. They went over to Lisa Spencer's and now me.

I said to Mike, "I thought you were going to your dad's."

"Oh, I didn't have to, or I'm going later," he said.

Then Mike said he was going to walk over to Mark Kaplan's, and Joe begged to use the bathroom. So finally I let him inside. When Mike was gone Joe said, you know why Mike didn't want to go with you? He just didn't want to. He never did. He was never going to go. How could you have thought he'd go with you? You're such a prude. He never liked you, and I never did either. You think I was serious when I said everything to you this summer? That was a whole game with Mike and me to see how far you'd go along.

I said, "That's not true about you. I just hurt you and now you're trying to hurt me by saying all this."

"But," he said, "you'll never really know that, will you? You'll never really know. Ha-ha."

It's the first time I'm writing without good news. I mean I'm not actually depressed, or am I? Nothing seems right. I'm shaky with everything, boys, friends, even family and me. I know eventually something will happen, but I just don't know when. *I will lose the weight and look and feel terrific.* I gained six pounds. I can't believe it. This has really pushed me over the limit, 126 pounds! God, I can't take this. Now that it's written that I'll lose it, it's set. I think I'll just remember, "We can take forever a minute at a time." My philosophy now. The summer will be nice. Joining the tennis club like everyone else on the team would have been. Oh well, no sense fighting a losing battle, I thought, but then my dad said we are joining! Jim Stern's junior prom seems like a long time ago. Very interesting. I think I must have let out a huge sigh when Jim just hugged me. Maybe I was just a little disappointed. Nah, that's ultra-hypocritical! I guess I really am pretty special. I'll make it!

Up to this point, I have been writing sporadically. I would like to start putting my feelings on paper more frequently. I'm always fascinated when I look back at the entries—actually being able to recapture the emotions is great. I am writing this solely for me. Maybe I'll be able to see myself changing, growing, progressing.

I would like to lose weight and look and feel terrific. The question is, can I? Well, I guess anything's possible. I really do want to, but I'm afraid. I have this strange notion that every single problem I have will disappear with those pounds. What if they don't, or what if I work really hard, and I can't do it and I don't know why. I really have to go back to school as a different person. Last year wasn't the pits. Or was it?? I must do this, if for no one else, for me. I deserve the confidence it will give me. Some people might not think that being 5'4" and weighing 126 is a lot, but I know it is!

I want to write about something that I have trouble admitting even to myself. The way I eat is definitely weird! I'm not always sure why I do it. All I know is, *I must stop.* If I don't, what will my future be? When I live alone, it'll be too easy. I'll be a blimp. Do I need help? I really don't think so. I mean, I'm not sick! Well, that's just it, I'm quitting cold turkey. Tonight will be the test, babysitting. Oh, God, when I think back to every Saturday night for years, eating like a pig! The candy, the soda, the cookies, the ice cream, all the things we never had at home and were encouraged not to eat. How many times did I eat and eat and eat and then run around the house while the kids slept doing push-ups, sit-ups, jumping jacks, anything to erase the Oreos, the Ding Dongs, the cans of Coke, the TV dinners? How many times did I stare at myself in the bathroom mirror wondering how many pounds I had gained, anxious for tomorrow when I could start fresh and, hopefully, not eat at all.

I'm fed up with myself! Why am I starting to cry? Because it's true, I want to change. I guess I *can* do anything! Well, I can't go on like this. I hate myself when I do it. I hate myself! I want to like myself. *I will.*

I felt really, really depressed and sad on my year anniversary with Joe, my first boyfriend. I don't know why. I remembered everything. Everything about Joe, and about Joe and Mike came flooding back.

Talking to Krista Jennings at the barbecue on Saturday, I realized that even though I'm as straight as the shortest distance between two points (straighter), I wouldn't want to be like her for anything. I wonder a lot if I'm normal. I can't stand the taste of alcohol, even wine. I know I never will. I've never had even one drink in my entire life. I'm not at all curious to even try marijuana, or any drugs, or smoking—even once.

Some world, you have to wonder if it's abnormal to be a totally logical thinking, sensible, healthy, sane, sober, intelligent person.

Well, I'll keep you updated on my progress, and anytime I feel weak, I'll write instead of eat.

JULY 8

Official Contract

Lisa Dale Messinger does hereby swear never to binge again. *Never.* I realize that this is in my best interest, and my best interest *is* my best interest!

I love *me!*

Signed,
Lisa Dale Messinger

JULY 10

Nobody's awake, but I've had a revelation! All I have to do to weigh 115 by August 31 is to lose a quarter of a pound a day! I can do that! That's one pound every four days. Maybe, if I'm good, I can even lose more! This really gives me confidence! Even if I have, by cheating spells, gone up to 128, I can still lose 13 pounds in 52 days. Isn't that great! It makes it seem so much more attainable. Wow. I guess this is positive thinking!

JULY 18

Meal Ticket Exchanges
(According to my nutritionist)

Breakfast:
1 cup nonfat milk
1 fruit
1 bread
1 meat (optional)
1 tsp. fat

Lunch:
vegetables (free)
1 fruit
1 bread
2 meats
1 tsp. fat

Snack:
(two out of three)
1 fruit
1 bread
1 meat

Dinner:
1 cup nonfat milk
vegetables (free)
1 fruit
1 bread
3 meats
1 tsp. fat

JULY 31

I am so *proud!* It's 1:26 A.M. I can't sleep so I'm trying on clothes. Guess who just zipped up that previously-given-up-on white skirt and guess who doesn't look that shabby in her size-five dressy pants that didn't fit six months ago? Hallelujah!

Two weeks with my nutritionist and I don't believe it. Slowly but *surely* I'm disappearing. I'm so glad Mom told me about her friend who was seeing this nutritionist and asked if I would want to go. It's the *real me* that's beginning to appear!

Keep up the good work!

SEPTEMBER 23

Could it be magic? Right now, I'm really not sure. You'll be one of the first to know if it is. Chris seems fantastic to me, but looks and personality aren't everything. Well, I shouldn't get my hopes up, Ellen did meet him first and does have two classes with him. I'll just have to play it by ear. I wish . . . well, I'm surviving better than ever before. I've got more friends now and am happy, with or without Mr. Right!

By seeing the nutritionist this summer (and still going), at this, the start of my junior year, I've lost at least $14\frac{1}{2}$ pounds. I weigh about 116. People say I really look thin. I still need a little convincing. If this situation with Chris works out I'll be shocked.

NOVEMBER 17

Lisa Messinger will weigh 115 pounds.

Lisa Messinger will accomplish this by December 4.

Lisa Messinger does swear, on my honor, to eat sensibly from this day forward.

After each "balanced" meal a penny will be put in a jar.

My reward upon completion will be—assuming that said weight has been maintained for three weeks, until 25 December, (during this period every "balanced" meal will warrant a nickel)—a $150.00 wardrobe.

I do hereby swear that I comprehend and will uphold the terms laid out in this contract.

Officially,
Lisa Messinger

DECEMBER 31

New Year's Resolutions

✔ Think positive thoughts about myself.

✔ Keep weight and figure at a point where I am happy about myself.

✔ Be happy.

✔ Be neater.

✔ Be confident.

Lisa Messinger does hereby swear to uphold these vows.

Signed sincerely,
Lisa Messinger

JANUARY 21

Well, it's the last day of my sixteenth year. I'm looking forward to getting older, being able to do more things and meet more people. Right now I'm very close to Cheri and (good friends, too, with) her boyfriend Todd. *I wish I had a boyfriend.* I know the mature attitude is just to wait for "my time to come." But I can't help wondering what it would be like to love someone, or at least really like them a lot and feel comfortable with them. I would not count Allan as a boyfriend (although he'd probably disagree). Just because we go out a lot doesn't mean we're a couple. He's nice and he's smart and he wants to be a reporter, but that's it. I don't want anything more with him.

Maybe I'm searching for something that doesn't exist. Oh, well. I still lack confidence in myself. I start building it up tomorrow!

I'm all right, I suppose.

FEBRUARY 13

Wish me luck. Tomorrow is Valentine's Day, and I am going to follow my heart. I have a good feeling inside that I've finally found someone who's good for me. Shyness on both parts, however, can definitely be a deterrent.

Even though Todd and Cheri are both very nice, apart and together, what they have would not be right for me. It's too intense. Maybe I'm on the brink of a relationship. Maybe not. Perry certainly is handsome. He certainly is. There's not much doubt there. *Very* intelligent too. So logical. And thinks like I do about so much. So easy to talk to, that is, when we have a real opportunity to talk. My feelings are right. I know it. This time it's special. Tomorrow my life might change. That's exciting. I'm not used to making a move like this. Although, I guess most people wouldn't consider giving a boy a Valentine's Day card such a big move. It's just that it's such a special recipient!

Keep that nerve up!

FEBRUARY 14

P.M.
So I didn't have the nerve. What else is new?

FEBRUARY 17

News Director
CBS Television, Los Angeles

Dear Mr. Short:

My reasons for writing are two-fold. First, I am seventeen years old and intent on becoming a broadcast journalist. I have taken broadcasting classes in school and have gotten experience on the local level. However, the real catalyst to my decision was the day I spent as one of your reporter's "shadow" for the TV newscast taping. After seeing the two of you and the rest of the news team at work, I was hooked. This brings me to my first question: Why aren't teens represented on TV? Although a few shows are directed toward young people, they are hosted by adults. Teenagers are apparent in other areas, from idolized actors to imprisoned criminals.

I would like to help break this barrier by appearing on your news magazine as one of the weekly guest hosts you advertised for on TV. My story idea deals with a serious, tragic and, too often, fatal issue that affects teens, adults and society as well, teenage suicide. I am on the speech team at my school (last year I was a National Forensic League State Finalist) and my current oratory deals with this topic. Through my research and interviews, I have become deeply concerned. Like most people, I was unaware of the great depth of this problem.

Trent Broadcasting Company
5th Avenue · New York, NY

Lisa Messinger
7089 Cardinal Drive
Encino, CA 91365

Dear Lisa,

As a producer for "K.I.D. NETWORK" I've received a letter
from you stating that you would like to appear as a news
reporter on our show.

To be a reporter for "K.I.D. NETWORK," you have to send us a
letter with an idea for a story from your neighborhood that
we would be able to film with you as a correspondent. This
story-idea should appeal to kids all over the country. If we
like the idea, we'll talk to you about it.

If you want to write us back with an idea, please include
a picture of yourself. Please also let us know your age
and telephone number.

Thanks from the "K.I.D. NETWORK."

Sincerely,

Jerry Dawber

Jerry Dawber
Executive Producer

Consider the statistics I've enclosed. What can we do about it? Many experts believe a broad educational effort is needed, that schools and suicide prevention centers should be combined in an effort to squelch the "epidemic."

My exposé could be filmed at a suicide prevention center. An opening would explain the gravity of the problem. I could then interview a teen who has attempted suicide, and a suicide expert who could give possible explanations and solutions.

Teen suicide is still sometimes a taboo subject. Only when we eliminate the myths can the problem be dealt with effectively.

Your TV show can help to inform the public, and, at the same time, give a future broadcaster her first break!

Thank you,
Lisa Messinger

FEBRUARY 23

John Arco
News Director
ABC Television, Los Angeles

Dear Mr. Arco:

Thank you for responding so quickly to my previous letter. I was very excited to learn that you had considered the idea of a teenage reporter, and would take the time to view my audition tape. It all goes to show that your open-mindedness and philosophy of there being more to life than news, weather, and sports is more than just talk. My response has been delayed because I have had trouble obtaining my original tape. During this interval, I have made an additional tape. I would greatly appreciate it if I could enhance my presentation with a personal meeting.

Becoming a broadcast journalist is my dream. As Helen Keller once said, "Follow your dreams, for as you dream you shall become."

Thank you very much for reading my letters and for taking a sincere interest in the concerns of your viewers.

Thank you,
Lisa Messinger

MARCH 12

I am very displeased with myself. I am fat! I am fat! I am fat! I hate myself! Maybe I'm not really fat, but, if that's how I feel, then there's really not much difference. I must change. I know I've said it before. I do not want to be as fat as I was last summer. One hundred thirty pounds. No way. With each pound it'll be harder!

If I begin now (and I know how to do it, too, because of going to the nutritionist last summer) then by this summer, I should be all set! If I could like myself in a bathing suit, that would be real progress! I must begin to feel more secure.

I suppose I'm like clay. I can leave myself in a blob or mold myself into a work of art.

MARCH 22

Spring will bring the turning over of a new leaf and a new life.

APRIL 3

Dear Congressman:

I have long had a dream of the ideal way to spend time a year from now, the summer following my high school graduation. I would consider it a privilege and an invaluable experience to have the opportunity to serve as a page in Congress. I understand the necessary qualifications, academic prowess, favorable recommendations, and corresponding interests. I feel that I fulfill these requirements. I have maintained a 4.0 grade average and am ranked first in my class. I was valedictorian at my junior high school graduation. I am extremely interested in politics, and am seriously considering the field as a future endeavor. My other possible career goals include broadcast journalism and law. My interests are related to these fields. As a freshman, I was editor-in-chief of our school newspaper. Incidentally, one of the highlights of my year as editor was an interview with you! In addition, I have been a member of the forensics and debate team for the past three years. During this time I have participated in a number of student congresses. In these the speakers play the part of congressmen attempting to pass legislation. I have learned a great deal through these experiences and I would love to have the chance to observe the real-life model of our enactments. I have greatly enjoyed these speech experiences and was proud to be one of the first three students to represent our high school at the State Forensics Finals in San Diego earlier this month. I have been reading about the duties and life style of a Congressional page, and the more I learn the more enthusiastic I become. I have included applicable recommendations and would gladly furnish any other necessary information.

I would consider it a privilege to speak or meet with you in the future.

Thank You,
Lisa Messinger

(Never Sent)

JUNE 28

I have to take this hostessing job. It will help me. You can't be shy when your job is to help people, to smile, to chat, to direct to a table. I'll have to do it. It'll be my job.

And in the more real world, I'll just be me. No grades. Just me. If I'm pretty, I'm pretty. If I'm smart, I'm smart.

This will help me become not shy, which I know I must become.

JULY 18

Wow. Did I expect this? This is okay. Here I am out in the real world, and I'm finally being noticed a little bit. My favorite, (twentyeight), sits at the counter and asks me out on dates! And he's not the only one who says things.

Maybe my parents have been right, maybe I am pretty. From what they say, these guys seem to think so, too, and I weigh 120.

JULY 20

I think...
I know that I think . . .
I think that I know . . .
I think that I know what I think . . .
I know what I know . . .
I think?

AUGUST 1

What are you doing? List it, then maybe you'll see:

- strawberry shortcake
- cream of potato soup
- chocolate pudding
- chocolate sauce
- cheddar cheese soup
- cream of chicken soup

You're supposed to be the take-out girl. Stop taking out to the bathroom or home! Stop it!

AUGUST 20

Well, I hope I'm not jumping the gun again! I've thought so many times that something was going to happen between us and I've been wrong, and we've just stayed friends. I really feel like this time it could be different though. I get a funny feeling in my stomach. Could it be love? No, now you are jumping ahead. Take your time. Don't blow it! Will Perry call? He will. He said so! I know he likes me. I just know it. You don't talk like that to someone you don't like. But how much? I wonder what's going to happen. I guess I have to make it happen.

Well, I feel good and that's good. 120 pounds is a nice round number. Pardon, a nice slim number, and still losing. I won't blow that again. So am I pretty? Sometimes I think so. Sometimes not. Enough people say so. Why always the *wrong* people?

Well, Perry's call just came and so did more doubts. Everything I just said about us might be void. Might be!

```
CBS News
524 West 57 Street
New York, New York 10019

Dear Ms. Messinger:

Thank you for your interest in our teen news program.
I think you summed it up when you said that the adult hosts
are serious journalists. Indeed they are with considerable
experience behind them. That was our first consideration in
selecting the hosts for this broadcast. I'd like to be able
to give you a chance, but before you could be considered
you would have had to already shown the type of journalism
background and talent which is the hallmark of CBS News.
     Good luck.

     Yours truly,

     Joel Heller
     Joel Heller, Executive Producer
```

SEPTEMBER 1

Perry,

This is a message that comes with the hope that you will *finally* get the message! You're so smart and quick-minded that it's really very surprising that it takes you so long to figure out such a simple little thing. Or maybe you have already figured it out? I know this is resorting to a pretty juvenile, junior-highish mode of communication, but I don't know what else to do. If you would just cooperate, it would all be so simple! Now here's my plan. (You have a relatively easy part.) Just come to me and say, "I have something I want to tell you." Then I'll say, "Don't say another word. I understand." Eight little words from you that have a big meaning. Oh, what's the point? I'll never have the nerve. As if I ever did!

2. I'll Diet 'Til I Drop

17 TO 18 YEARS OLD

Bust: 35"

Upper leg: 23"

Waist: 27$\frac{1}{4}$"

Lower leg: 12$\frac{1}{2}$"

Hips: 37"

Midriff: 35"

Calf: 8"

Lower arm: 8$\frac{1}{4}$"

Upper arm: 13"

Almost eighteen. Almost an adult. Almost grown-up. Almost out on my own. "Almost" seems to be the story of my life. I feel kind of out of it this year. You know, the awkward year. The in-between one. I keep wondering where I'll be and what I'll be doing next year. If I had to guess (and wish), I'd say I'll be at UCLA living in the dorm. I'd be surprised if I were in an apartment or at home, and even more surprised if I were at another school.

This year I just can't get into anything, my classes, the tennis team or the speech team. My interest level seems to have disappeared. That's about the state of my love life too, non-existent. Sometimes I wonder if there are any other normal acting, intelligent people who are as inexperienced in the field of sex as I am. With things like smoking and drugs I have absolutely no interest. Drinking I just plain dislike. But sex, if I found the right person I would like to try. Maybe not the whole banana, but I'd certainly like to get a little experience behind me.

Well, I did one good thing. I joined a health club. I wonder if by next year it will have paid off?

Oh, Prince Charming, come out, come out wherever you are! Or at least send one of your friends to keep me occupied until you get here.

Perry, I just give up. Not that I tried all that hard. But you're much too shy (I hope), and I can't, no matter how much I think about it, make that first move.

It just seems like nothing very important is happening to me. Or maybe I just don't notice it. Maybe this is life.

OCTOBER 22

Happy birthday to me! Happy birthday to me! Oh, I know I'm exactly three months off. But I've already decided on a present to myself: a new me, and I've got three whole months to deliver. It won't stop there, and I won't sluff off in the meantime. I am in the process of creating a more beautiful me through proper nutrition and exercise. Oh, I can just imagine me three months from now.

Maybe I can even do it before. At any rate, it *will* happen, and afterward it will be my way of life!!

OCTOBER 30

There's, of course, going to be no way I'm going to go to UCLA now. They don't even have a journalism major there, let alone a broadcast journalism major.

No, I have seen my school. Thank God I competed in a speech tournament there. USC. "The ghetto," my mother always said. What a picture I had of it in my mind. Ha! This school is beautiful.

Somehow I know that when I look in my high school counseling center's college catalogs, I will find a broadcast journalism major at USC. At my school.

NOVEMBER 13

Day One (Of thirty days spent following Overeaters Anonymous diet with an O.A. sponsor)

Breakfast:
1 egg
1 oz. cheddar cheese
1 apple
tea with artificial sweetener

Lunch:
4 oz. tuna fish
1 serving cooked carrots
finger salad with lettuce
(Make sure it's all right to have lettuce in a finger salad.)
diet soda

Dinner:
4 oz. turkey without skin
1 serving string beans
2 cups salad with diet dressing
diet soda

Finally, I have met people I can talk to at Overeaters Anonymous.

Go at night, spill out your guts, come home, and lie again. Keep the truth hidden.

The strongest feeling I had at O.A., though, was fear and shock. Older people, like in their 40s or 60s, were talking about the same compulsive eating problems that I have.

Somehow I always imagined that this ended. I never pictured having this in college or, especially, in later life. I'm going to have a tremendously successful career and life and marriage. I never pictured this. I always thought that it would just go away when I got out of high school.

Well, now I'm scared to death and more determined to get out of this thing soon, because I see in her eyes and hers and hers and his and his and hers that it doesn't just end. I can't waste my life, not *my* life.

DECEMBER 14

Dear, dear Lisa,

You are such a beautiful person to have shared your most private feelings with me in the hopes that you could in some way help me.

You are very dear to me Lisa and I feel that you do know it, but it is still too soon in our relationship for you to fully know the scope of all you mean to me.

I cried and cried over all the love that spilled from your words on those sheets of paper and shall reread them many times over. I have already read your letter about fifteen times.

I know all your feelings because I have felt them all *from a very young age until today*. I also think I know the answers now. However, knowing and *doing something about it* are two entirely different areas. You don't have to let food get you down. You can control your life. The problem can be conquered, corrected, and permanently erased in your case because you are so young, and "NOW IS THE TIME."

I only hope that when Vicki and I move to California (I can't believe you were only two years old the last time I saw you) we can have long talks, and I can give you the benefit of my experiences and help you so that you will *at long last* learn to like Lisa and appreciate her for the beautiful human being she is.

Eating is only a symptom. The cause is much deeper.

I must admit I am a little discouraged. I have reached a plateau after losing twelve pounds and still feel huge. I try to walk at lunchtime, but it is not always easy to get out. One of the girls is out of the office, etc., that kind of thing. At night it is dark. I will have to try and find a way. I am doing above the waist exercises daily and they seem to be helping somewhat.

All I can say is, keep up the good attitude, exercise, and much love to you. I am so grateful you found out that I was in Overeaters Anonymous in New York and knew that your own California Overeaters Anonymous experience would make us soul mates. I would make this longer, but I finally want to get it into the mail.

Much love always honey,
Aunt Judith

DECEMBER 16

I guess I have to let things happen to actually believe that they are possible. I suppose that's why I gained back the weight that I lost last summer. I had to show myself that I could put it back on.

I guess that's why I had to take that one bite. I didn't believe that I would not be able to stop. After that first jellybean, man, that was it. So, I guess you learn by trial and error. Well, now that I truly believe that I do have a disease, maybe I can begin to cure it.

As they say in O.A., *without exception,* abstinence is the most important thing in my life!

DECEMBER 20

The first page of one of my many blank writing journals.

This collection of thoughts is hereby dedicated to:

- The new me.
- The product of all my hopes and dreams.
- The contented person that I, in due time, *will* become.

The first entry in the new journal, written that same day:

I am going to give myself a present. I can't say it is for my eighteenth birthday, although, of course, it is. I can't say it's for Christmas or Hanukkah, but it is. I can't say it's given in the spirit of the New Year, but a sense of beginnings is a part of it. I can't say it's a graduation present, although I am graduating on more than one level.

My present is, in a sense, in celebration of all these occasions. But to work it's got to be much more than that. I am giving myself my life. Control of it. Pride in it. The joy of living it day to day. I was going to say that I'm giving myself back my life. But then I realized that I'm not at all sure that I ever really had it.

I want it. Losing weight is only a tool that I will use to find the happiness and confidence that is in store for me. Before I will be able to see clearly, I will have to wipe away the clouds. When I am thin, I will be able to deal objectively and realistically with the true problems. I am unable to do that now.

I know that I can do it. I need to if I want to keep my sanity.

Happy New Year
Happy Birthday
Merry Christmas
Happy Hanukkah
Happy Graduation
Happy Tomorrows
Fulfilled Today

West Valley High School
Abuela School District

Office of Principal
The Parent Faculty Club
Music Boosters

To Whom It May Concern:

I would like to take this opportunity to recommend Lisa
Messinger, currently a senior at our high school, as a student
of the highest caliber and potentially a great addition to the
student body of the University of Southern California (USC).

As Lisa's counselor, I have watched her progress over four
years and it would be difficult for me to imagine any student
having as fine a high school career as Lisa has had. In terms of
academic accomplishment, Lisa has maintained a straight A (4.0)
average in a difficult and demanding program. Additionally,
she has exemplified herself in the area of speech and has won
the outstanding student award at our school.

Having taught Lisa in the classroom, I can speak with
authority when I say that Lisa exemplifies the best qualities
of scholarship and academic enthusiasm.

However, Lisa's academic abilities are only a part of
what makes her such a fine candidate. Even more important are
Lisa's personal qualities. She displays a concern for others
and maturity uncommon in people her age, and is able to
interact successfully with all types of people. Additionally,
Lisa has a fine sense of humor and is able to keep life in
perspective.

Recently, Lisa has decided on a tentative career choice in
the field of broadcasting. Her exceptional verbal abilities and
ease with people lead me to believe that this is an appropriate
choice for her. Hopefully, you will be able to see the
excellence we see in Lisa and will accept her into your program.

Thank you.

Richard First

Richard First
Counselor

JANUARY 4

I made an appointment for a tour guide interview at Universal Studios (que sera sera).

I get spurts of energy and then they fade. I'm going to pick up the energy level of my lifestyle. Running? Maybe? It's neat out there before the sun, peaceful (but early)!

The high price of my impending college education is beginning to worry me.

JANUARY 5

It's one minute at a time. And this minute, 12:19 P.M., I feel happy. So I guess for the moment I've got everything I want.

Something I read, and thought might be a morale booster, "Remember that the only thing that stands between you and success is you. Resolve to accept life as it comes and make the best of it, knowing that by doing so, you create an even better tomorrow."

JANUARY 6

Size seven. Size seven. Size seven. Here I am in Palm Springs and I am wearing size seven purple pants. Corduroy to be exact. And a beautiful mauve sweater. What are hours of dressing and make-up when it can turn out like this?

I have been kissed by a football player. A college football player. A rugged, curly haired, adorable football player. With a gorgeous physique.

Pecked, yes. Really kissed, no. Why did I turn my cheek? I dance with him all night, even after my parents leave the hotel club, and then I turn my cheek. What is wrong with me? I was all ready for a tongue. I saw him coming at me outside my hotel room. I saw the mouth open. I saw the tongue. I thought, "This guy's 19. This time I'm gonna do it. No touchy, no feely, just the tongue." And I didn't.

But I don't really care, because I'm getting out of my purple pants and I'm going to sleep and I'm really not the least bit unhappy!

JANUARY 10

Here I stand at the crossroads of my life. I am at an ending and a beginning. I am at a vital point.

I look back. I see years of disgust, anguish, insecurity, tears, unfulfillment.

I know that I am about to embark on an exciting, lifelong journey. I am packing my mental bags and am on the brink of moving on. As I look ahead I see the first rays of sunshine and in the distance a rainbow.

I know that once I take that first step there is no turning back, my life will begin.

I am scared, but here I go. One quick glance back, and a sigh of relief. Life, here I come.

JANUARY 12

Lisa's New Life!

Meal Plan

Breakfast:
1 fruit
1 bread
1 meat
1 fat

Lunch:
vegetables (unlimited)
1 fruit
1 bread
2 meats
1 fat

Snack:
1 fruit

Dinner:
vegetables (unlimited)
1 fruit
1 bread
3 meats
1 fat

No switching around of foods. Always eat at same place when at home. Keep a food diary.

Exercise Program

Jogging: Every morning. Start at two times around block. Progress as ready.

Home Work Out: Once each day, after school.

Health Club Exercise Class: Every day! Preferably the 6:30 P.M. class.

Shopping Mall Ice Skating: One hour each weekday. Preferably from 12:00–1:00 P.M.

Tennis: Once on Sundays. During the week, as much as possible.

Bike Riding: Once on Sundays for at least one hour and five miles.

JANUARY 16

I smiled before I went to sleep tonight. I know tomorrow is going to be a bright and beautiful day, a new chance that will bring me closer to my new life.

JANUARY 24

What in the hell is the matter with me? This is supposed to be my new life. It's already working, somewhat. I look pretty good. I feel pretty good.

However, a one-pound bag of peanut M&M's, Miss Messinger, is not in your new life plan. No. No. No. Why the hell did you eat them? Sure, they were for your eighteenth birthday party tonight. Right. Your parents have already bought enough food for thirty more people than the thirty who have been invited. You were supposed to be taking your SAT's, not be on a sugar high.

Granted, a 4.0 GPA may not force you to perform magnificently on SAT's, but a sugar rush and shaking hand do not make great test takers.

What the hell is the matter with you? You are doing okay, and, bam, you're flat on your back. Shape up.

JANUARY 30

"Would you care to join me in the bathroom?" Not your run-of-the-mill question. However, I assure you it was prompted more out of desperation than a desire for companionship. The party was ending. My eighteenth birthday party gala was almost "kaput," as was any chance for my romantic future. You see, Perry Schwartz was about to walk out the door taking all of my starry-eyed dreams with him.

I had to do something. It was now or never. I opted for the now. That's when I dragged him into the bathroom, our only place of refuge. In his eyes, was that the desire I had so often dreamed of, or was it just fear? We've all heard tales of love-starved women attacking innocent young men in deserted powder rooms.

At any rate, I popped the question. And, after a slight deliberation, he popped the answer, he would be "honored" to escort me to the school's Sadie Hawkins' Dance. Dreams come true. Wishes are granted. Prayers are answered. The boy of my dreams, quite literally, was interested, semi-interested, or, at least, showed a flicker of interest.

I had plotted, planned, mapped out, lived out that moment a thousand times in my imagination. In fact, it was that playacting that gave me courage and confidence. Well, what I lacked in courage and confidence, I made up for in adrenaline.

Now, I'm a firm believer in the power of illusion. I'm also a firm believer in the power of pine-scented Lysol. I'm really not quite sure which did the trick.

JANUARY 30

Dear Lisa,

Just a word of thanks for inviting me to your birthday party. I really enjoyed myself, as I am sure everyone else did as well. I am really glad I went and am looking forward to seeing you again soon.

Love,
Perry

FEBRUARY 24

Wow! That's about the only adjective that truly describes my feelings. Or maybe devastated. I think I'm in shock or a tailspin or something. I have certainly never felt this way before. It's a layman's guess, but I think I may be in love. I don't believe it. That's the first time I've admitted it even to myself. How come after all of this time knowing each other things seem to be happening so fast? I feel so inexperienced. The fact that Perry probably is too doesn't console me. He seems to catch on fast.

God! He likes me. After all of this time, it doesn't seem real! I have never been so nervous and reacted in such a way. The pains in my stomach have been unreal. They almost work as a sexual alarm system.

Sex? Hmmmm. It crossed my mind last night that he could be *the* first. But I trust him and his judgment so much.

Because I want it to work so much, I get too tense. Before the Sadie Hawkins' Dance tonight nothing. Now, he's kissed me about eight times (count 'em, eight!). I kissed him once. And, brother, if holding my hand can make me go limp, I don't know what the big stuff is going to do. His arms around me slow dancing close . . . I like it all. I'm afraid, scared. He's so sweet and *handsome*. Everything I see I like.

I wonder how he's feeling. Talking abstractly a few weeks ago, as friends only, we both said we didn't want to get involved with anyone right now, but, of course, that wasn't quite true on my part! And it seems like it might not have been truth on his part, either! And now, regardless of that, it's on such a personal level.

What next? I am so confused! (But it's a nice kind of confusion.)

MARCH 20

I am very happy! All of those times I thought I was on the verge of something, and nothing! Then all of a sudden happiness crept up on me!

I've never looked or felt better. I think I am in love with Perry. If it isn't, it's the closest I've ever come.

I've grown up . . . in more ways than one!

I really am happy!

MARCH 21

Well. Well. Well. You know that experience I wanted behind me, it's behind me. I must say I think my sexual attitude is very healthy.

Although the Big Event hasn't been staged yet, I feel as though I know more about it.

It was right. It was natural. I would say I love Perry but I am not sure what love is.

What I do know is that I feel more deeply, and care more about him, and really truly like him more than anyone I've ever met.

So, whatever happens I will not regret last night. It was part of my growing up cycle. It is a part of my adult life.

MARCH 24

Have I been taking things for granted? Maybe I shouldn't trust my judgment so much. This is all so new to me. I don't want to make a wrong move. Perry has never told me how he feels. I mean in three words or less: i.e., "I love you." "I like you." "Bug off." Of course, he has said he likes me. No shit! (I'm getting vulgar in my old age.) Well, my mom said that my dad wouldn't say it for a long time either, and look at them, they've been married almost 30 years. I don't know if I am in love or not, but I like the way I am feeling. Although, today I am a little anxious. I wonder if all his thinking will amount to "Take a hike." No, he wouldn't hurt me. Intentionally, that is. At all costs, the relationship is worth it. Now that I've finally got something special, I'm not giving up so easily. Turn of thought: I surprise myself. My attitude about sex had always been liberal, but abstract. Now the situation is personal. I can't believe how comfortable I was. It felt right. It is right.

I am so grateful that I don't have any hang-ups about this all-important part of life. (Hope he doesn't.)

Grateful, too, to my wonderful mom who makes it so easy. She must be one in a million. He is too. So am I.

You know, I was just thinking all of this is important, but what's really important is how I feel about myself. And even though I ate like a maniac today (insecurity), I like myself. I am worthwhile. I am a good person. I have a lot of added extra-special qualities. I'll make it. I forgive myself (for eating). If that isn't progress!

I love myself. God, I think I've just had an experience comparable to any "born again" experience. Better. Live!

Later

I eat to escape. Is it possible that I just realized this? Could I be that dense? Didn't I know it all the time? Shove in the food, turn on the TV and tune out; that's the pattern. Now that I'm eighteen, I can write my own excuse notes for school. Escape notes. Do the Winchell's donut run (1 dozen assorted), get the Haagen-Dazs (a pint of mint chocolate), a few cans of Coke and lie down in front of the soap operas in the guest room. Parents at work. Door closed. Just stay outside, Consuela. Don't clean in the guest room today or two days from now or next Tuesday. Lisa is occupying the guest room, Consuela.

MARCH 26

I just received my housing confirmation from USC. Soon my whole life will be dramatically changing (starting). I am looking forward to college life, but right now ain't so bad either. Whether I'm in love or not is not important. I am comfortable in a relationship (with a capital "R," as Perry so cutely put it). I am learning about life and about myself. I feel lucky to have someone so compatible and likable. Physically speaking, it is amazing how quickly I have adapted. I like it (which I never thought I would), but am not overcome with the heat of passion (which is what I thought would happen). Keeping control is no problem. I am comfortable. I think that somewhere out there is someone who will spark my passion, emotional and physical, and then I will know love. But for now I am content. For once, I am at the right place at the right time.

10:40 P.M.

Whew! I feel 100 percent better. Revived. Invigorated. Awake. Alive again. Boy, exercise really does make a difference. While I was in bed I was thinking, I can't wait until tomorrow to get back on track after blowing it today by overeating. Then I thought, I could still get something done tonight. I'm glad I did. Wow, I didn't go Saturday, Sunday, Monday, Tuesday or Wednesday, didn't lift a muscle. I felt awful, tired, cranky. Now I feel better. I shouldn't bite the hand. This health club really shaped me up. I shouldn't slack off, or it'll be Flabsville! I think I'll dance a bit before bed. Exercise is where it's at.

11:06 P.M.

Well, I just danced around like crazy and I feel great. This is the *best* therapy. It really is an attitude reverser. Before, I felt lazy and fat like I wouldn't be able to get back into it. Well, I did great. I want to do my workout again before bed.

Tomorrow, here I come!

MARCH 27

My Food Plan

Breakfast:		Lunch:	
1 bread	70	1 bread	70
1 meat	90	2 meats	130
1 fruit	60	1 fat	40
	220	veggies	free
			240

Dinner:

1 bread	70	**Total:**	700 calories
2 meats	130		
1 fat	40		
veggies	free		
	240		

MARCH 30

Well, well, well. If I didn't know better, I'd say Perry is most definitely in love with me. But, of course, I know better. I'm not ruling out the possibility, though. What the hell? Why label it? The feelings are great! He cares. I care. We're both lucky, two prudes in a pod *quickly* adapting!

I forgive myself. I've got a lot going for me. Why blow it by eating?

MARCH 31

1:31 A.M.
Alone in house. Perry just left. Feel fine. A real make-out artist. I like it. No passion. Well, maybe a little bit.

APRIL 5

I am finally alone. There is, finally, something so personal I will not tell. It is my decision. My choice. Not Perry's. Not Mom's. Mine. Right now, I feel that I will abstain. Of course, I reserve the right to change my mind. First, because he's not said he loves me. But he does. If he were madly in love with me, I would. But he's not that type. I love him, but I'm not madly in love either.

What we have is very special. It doesn't come along every day. Some people never find it. We are lucky. However, I will not risk pregnancy, and even with every precaution there is still that possibility. Right now, it's just not worth it to either of us.

How do I feel? I feel capable, normal, a little aggressive. I guess I'll just have to take life one day at a time.

Good idea.

APRIL 7

I feel so lucky. I have such a wonderful boyfriend, such an open relationship. We feel the same way about so many important things. Sex. That's important. We are having a physical relationship. I've been wanting to say that. I feel so comfortable. However, not comfortable enough to go "all the way," although I can see how some girls could. He's got *some* build!

I am in love, in a way, but I don't know if I'm in love with Perry or with the idea of being in love. I have a feeling it's the latter. Oh well, I feel great. I never could understand what "making out" was. Needless to say I do now, and I like it. I really do. Shock!

If Rod Burke asked me out, would I go? Probably, since Perry made a point of saying no commitments.

I don't ever want to forget how I feel now. *Content!* A feeling relatively new to me.

APRIL 7

1:04 A.M.

I can't sleep. Maybe I drank too much diet soda today. I was hungry and had a craving for cereal (even my cravings are nutritious now), so I had a bowl. It's nice to be able to eat without blowing it. It's a good feeling to have some leeway. I must admit I've been feeling pretty wonderful lately, but it's a different kind of wonderful. I've been up and down, but the ups have been prevailing.

The prom is in fifty days. How nice to have someone so special at such a special time. He will ask me. (He'd better.) I know it will be a beautiful night, even better than the Sadie Hawkins' Dance, if that's possible. Grad night, too, will be a ball, a far cry from last year's with that jerk. I'll ask Perry to that, if time starts running out.

Perry is so handsome. Gorgeous, dark curly hair (which my fingers always end up running through). Beautiful (an understatement) green eyes. Dark, smooth complexion that's always tan. (No pimples!) Broad, broad shoulders. Arms with just the right kind of muscles. Cute, cute hairless chest (the best kind). Flat, hard stomach. Oops, I forgot those big, nicely curved lips and long, luscious tongue. And, of course, those huge, masculine hands. Sexy, sexy, tan, hairy, long, muscular legs. In other words, no complaints!

Understandably, the newness of romance has taken up much of my thoughts. I catch myself thinking about him a lot. Thinking is one thing, but I don't want to bore people. Boredom hasn't been a problem for me lately. I've been excited both mentally (he is the most intelligent person I know) and physically. Physically, I have been discovering quite a lot about myself. I am by no means inhibited. I am in control, but not inhibited, and very spontaneous— traits I thought I lacked, especially in this area. I like kissing a lot and everything else too. I think I will like "it" too, but *we* have decided not to get "totally" involved. I am satisfied with this decision.

Honestly, I am feeling more satisfied with most things lately. I'm finally living in the present, not contemplating the future and daydreaming about what college will be like. Believe it or not, I am happy with myself. I like the way I look. I really think 122 pounds is okay. This is not to say that I'm still not trying to improve. I am. The difference is that I'm not obsessed with losing weight, merely determined. I realize that what I've got is pretty good and I can only get better. I have not forgotten, though, that it is all too easy to slip and binge again, especially when overconfidence and the feeling that things have always been dandy sets in. This is not true. I've made myself miserable in the past. I'm walking a fine line, and it would be easier to fall than continue on the tightrope. This must always be in the back of my mind, that refraining from binging is a daily accomplishment.

I won't take it for granted.

What I went through to get Perry taught me that when you really want something you have to go for it. Then, once you get it, it takes hard work to keep the sailing smooth. But, it is *definitely* worth it!

APRIL 8

Wow! I'm really shaping up! All this going to the club after school and exercising on my own is finally paying off. My upper arm is smaller, so are legs. Stomach is pretty hard, face a bit thinner. Don't know what I weigh at the moment, probably about 121. That's okay, though I still want to lose.

God, do I have a handsome boyfriend! I have good taste. Today when Perry came over, whoa! He looked very sexy to me. Cha, cha, cha.

We've been kissing on the run lately, but it's fun, and the pecks have turned into flicks. I like.

I can't wait until the prom. *Boy,* am I happy.

APRIL 9

Forget the past.
Nothing is irreversible, not even eating 10,000 calories.
Life is an exciting adventure
That starts anew each day.
You've got it, so do something with it!

APRIL 11

I do not understand myself to say the least! So cocky, mentally that is. I fell from my tightrope.

Right now, I'm getting up and brushing myself (my ego) off. Or at least I think so. Who can say for sure? I know that I hate living in the pits, and I don't ever have to be there. I have control over it.

The bottom line is that I feel great when I abstain. Yes, abstain! That Overeaters Anonymous word. Ominous, but true. It's not being perfect or inflexible. It is abstaining from compulsive overeating. It's not worth it to let go and get flabby. I care too much about myself.

APRIL 15

I am happy. I could be miserable, but I'm not. I have such good friends. Perry is such a wonderful boyfriend! They all stuck up for me. Because of their support I didn't overeat to solve this problem with the speech team. A few people, according to my friends, can't stand me because I win and win and win on my own without selling my soul to the "group."

In terms of eating, past performance was forgotten. I didn't think about all of the times I did gorge to escape from these kinds of confrontations. I feel good about today. A potentially rotten experience turned out okay!

APRIL 18

I feel good! Perry, a wonderful boy, likes me. I feel like I'm in love, but who knows? I've felt like saying it, but I know I won't unless he does. He's so cute. We're so comfortable. We go together.

I like. I like. I like.

APRIL 19

Saturday 3:00 A.M.
I am definitely in love! I feel fantastic! This has been the best night of my life. Perry told me all he saw in me: pretty, brains, ambition, and asked me to the prom.

He feels for me! He loves me, I can tell. We won't say it yet, but someday. He's the most wonderful boy I ever met, and I love him.

Tonight was beautiful.

APRIL 25

I'm a very happy girl. It just dawned on me, I'm starting a weight loss program without being miserable and without being dumpy and bulgy. I'm happy and I look fine. What a switch, but it's that switch that will bring success. I know my goal, 110 pounds, and I will seek it realistically. I like what I'm starting out with, so I can only get better! What an attitude.

God, am I ever in love. I love love. This is terrific. Even when I'm down, I'm up. Perry's so right! Not perfect by any means, but that's what makes it so good and real, I know I haven't gone mushy. Well, I had my first bed experience. (Water yet!) It was a lot more comfortable than the couch, and especially the car. The prom is something to look forward to, but I like every day. They seemed numbered, like we're coming to the end of one life (high school) and the beginning of another (college). Could it be that we'll be the one overlapping link in each other's two lives?

What a beautiful thought.

APRIL 25

I am beginning a weight loss program. Seriously. My goal weight is 110 pounds. The program is 1,000 calories a day: three meals, one snack, or less.

Signed,

Lisa Messinger

(No frills this time.)

MAY 1

Weight: 122 pounds

Breakfast:

1 tbsp. peanut butter	90
2 slices thin bread	70
½ c. grapefruit juice	40
	200

Lunch:

tuna fish	90
diet mayo	40
1 bun	130
strawberries	30
	290

Snack:

yogurt	200

Dinner:

1 egg	90
1 regular bread	65
	155

Total: 845 calories

MAY 1

Bust: 36½"

Waist: 26½"

Hips: 36½"

Midriff: 34"

Upper arm: 10¼"

Upper leg: 21½"

Lower leg: 12½"

Calf: 8"

Lower arm: 8¼"

36½"—26½"—36½"

MAY 3

Saturday 5:41 A.M.

I think I'm confused. I don't know what the hell to think or do. One thing seems right, going out with only Perry. I also want to play the field, but I don't really want that. I was testing Perry. He said we should see other people as well as each other, and I said let's just keep seeing each other. He didn't back down and neither did I. Compromise. What happened to compromise? I guess you just can't compromise on some things. Why does he have to be so analytical and intelligent and logical?

God, *he thinks he's in love with me.* This is too much. And I said that I think I love him, too. He *can't* stop going out with me, even if he thinks we should see other people, too. *Love, love, love.* God, I want to be in love.

My first real orgasm. And I passed the bathing suit barrier. I actually wore one and got a compliment! I asked for it! Okay, okay, okay. Just take your time and think about it. This is GREAT!

MAY 5

Realizations: There are no more fat pockets on my legs ("beautiful" legs according to Perry, my beau). No more perpetual pimples. The ones that were always there . . . gone! Firm arms! No wishing, it just happened. No, I guess I did it.

Love . . . I'm in it.

What do I do? Take one day at a time. Remain calm. As they said, you're a calm person. Keep your calm! HE LOVES ME!

MAY 27

Bust: 36½"	Upper leg: 21½"
Waist: 26"	Lower leg: 12½"
Hips: 36"	Calf: 8"
Midriff: 33"	Lower Arm: 8¼"
Upper arm: 10¼"	

MAY 30—PROM DAY

WOW!
ME AND PERRY!!!
He couldn't keep his hands off me.
Hollywood hand-holding
Beach walking kisses
Beach blanket caresses
Jeremy's breakfast bash
Car in front of house under street light, me under him.

JUNE 6

Dreams can become realities.
Believe. Believe. Believe.
Not binging is not easy, but it's worth it!
You've come a long way, Baby!

JUNE 12

I've never felt better.

I didn't truly know Perry. He's so sincere. We compromised. We decided we could date other people as well as each other. After we made up, we went to the beach with Jeremy, Laura, and Glen. (Me at the beach in a teeny-weeny red bikini, that's what I call progress!)

JUNE 13—GRADUATION

Well, I was great! Not nervous giving the graduation speech at all. To me, this was a beautiful night. Everything was right, being with the Schwartz's and such a good friend like Leslie.

Grad night at Disneyland—well, I'll never look at "Small World" and "Haunted Mansion" in quite the same way. Perry couldn't seem to keep his hands off me on those rides or any other time, and I loved every minute of it. I couldn't keep my eyes off him. He looked so NICE. Such a NICE BOY.

Our little Swedish pancake breakfast party with our friends at my house was fun, but it's the "dessert" that I'll always remember.

What next? Will Perry and I end up together or apart? I'll just play it by ear.

Voted "Most Likely to Succeed." Boy, did I feel great (and surprised)!

JUNE 13

Dearest Lisa,

Hi! If you fall asleep over this I hope you find it and read it. I just want to tell you again how absolutely magnificent you were. You are beautiful (as always) and smart, witty, mature, and as I've thought always, too, "most likely to succeed." Well, what more could you ask for? Valedictorian, speeches, beautiful friends; you're a very lucky and successful girl. Now here's something I've never told anyone except you now, you are everything I utmost desire to be and achieve when I get older. Looks, brains, emotions, personality, all-around exceptional. You're a treasure to everyone you meet. Lately, I've felt close to you and I hope this summer holds more of that closeness in store for us. I wouldn't want to be in California (although I often have second thoughts about Mom and I having moved here) without someone like "specifically you," Lisa. I just wanted you to know how I felt. Although we vary a little in age, I still feel we have such good times together, and although your upcoming steps on life's winding roads will be tough ones, unique ones, remember I'll always be here and I'll always think of you *very often*. So take care because I love you so very much.

Love,
Vicki

JUNE 16

Sick and in bed. I think I'll write a few pages to a hypothetical autobiography:

Rob Jeffries was the boy voted Most Likely to Succeed in my senior class. He is your standard jockish, scholarly Aryan: baseball, football, and soccer varsity, and a 3.8 grade point average. He is rich, nice, and fairly straight. Voted Most Popular Boy and Prom King.

The girl voted Most Likely to Succeed should have been Kari Tamner. She was Associated Student Body President, nice, smart, blonde, and blue eyed. A four-year cheerleader, the only thing she had in common with the other cheerleaders was a great pair of legs. She is going to study communications at U.C., San Diego.

When I arrived at school on graduation morning, I was shocked to find out that Kari Tamner had not won and that I had. I was flocked by people I had barely spoken to in my four years of high school asking me why I had not been at the award's breakfast I had swept.

"God, you won Succeed, Best Public Speaker, and Best Student. Everyone was wondering where you were."

"Everyone" wondering where *I* was? I had been home in bed thinking how no one in the world, let alone the senior class, should give a damn about a worthless person like me.

I had gotten out of bed that morning, unlike so many mornings before, only because Dean Belgetti had said that if we didn't come to the final graduation rehearsal we wouldn't graduate. I, of course, lived by everything Dean Belgetti said, and besides, I was the graduation speaker.

On the mornings I didn't go to school, I'd stay home and watch soap operas, cry, and eat Winchell's donuts by the dozen, Haagen-Dazs ice cream by the pint, and Swanson TV dinners by the tray. It seemed like I spent half of my senior year in this manner. The other half I spent writing my own excuse notes (allowed once you were eighteen), and dropping courses right and left in order to preserve my status as a 4.0 student, not to mention my slot as valedictorian.

I was compulsive about those sorts of things, a perfectionist by birth. My mother tells me I cleaned my own diapers and burped myself. She may exaggerate, but I've taken over the exaggerating here. I've made my life one great big exaggeration.

Graduation day, by the way, was one of the best days of my life. Not because I graduated from high school and spent the night prancing around Disneyland with my boyfriend, but because I was succumbing to the tonsillitis and pink eye that would keep me drugged and dozing for the next several days. You see, when you're drugged and dozing you can't do much of anything, let alone eat. For the last several days I have subsisted on lemonade and popsicles.

Since my diet has consisted of more sugar than a sugar commercial, I thought I was gaining weight. You can imagine my surprise, therefore, when I stepped on the scale and saw in front of me the number 117, a virtual miracle. For most of my pubescent life I have hovered somewhere between 122 and 128 pounds. That is why graduation day was one of the best days of my life.

(To be continued, someday.)

How to Identify
an Eating Disorder

Lisa Messinger is the "every girl" who has come for help to my eating disorders psychotherapy practice for the last thirty years. From the moment I began reading Lisa's diary, as you probably were, too, I was drawn into her moving story. So, too, I am moved by my young clients who have the immediate ability to grab both my heart and soul, because—like Lisa—they are so very special. How can we use Lisa's story to help you or someone you love? I am honored to be able to possibly guide you or someone you care about in stopping this often life-threatening problem in its tracks. Through the essential information in this chapter that first defines the varied spectrum of eating disorders and then explains the medical, emotional, and behavioral symptoms—using stirring examples from Lisa's compelling diary to further clarify them—I have created a roadmap you can use to better steer yourself or someone you care about to safety.

Sometimes, people may not even realize that you need help. After all, as in Lisa's case, eating disorders usually attack the best and the brightest, people who are talented, attractive, sensitive, and "good." Like Lisa, people such as you or your loved one are often voted the most likely to succeed, best public speaker, and best student. But what has become startlingly apparent to me in my own practice is that these people, who on the surface seem to have everything and are easy for everyone to love, have already lost the ability to love themselves. Like in Lisa's case, often from a very early age, the self-loathing and destructive physical and emotional behaviors have begun.

Although eating disorders usually begin between the ages of about 12 and 24, like all eating-disorders professionals, I am seeing children as young as 9 in my practice (although eating disorders can certainly start in adulthood and even old age). Still a disease that primarily affects females, the number of males is continually rising.

Eating disorders are most insidious diseases. Many of you reading this book may already know only too well through your own experiences or those of a loved one just how true that statement is. As with Lisa, in most cases the disorder begins slowly and quietly, until, even before the person or anyone around them knows it, the disease has taken control, becoming serious, addictive, and potentially deadly. We have the privilege in this diary, caught on paper the moment it happened, of seeing how unassumingly it can begin.

"Nobody's awake," Lisa writes excitedly at 16 in one of her first journal entries ever about her weight, "but I've had a revelation! All I have to do to weigh 115 by August 31 is to lose a quarter of a pound a day! I can do that! That's one pound every four days. Maybe, if I'm good, I can even lose more! This really gives me confidence! Even if I have, by cheating spells, gone up to 128, I can still lose 13 pounds in 52 days. Isn't that great! It makes it seem so much more attainable. Wow. I guess this is positive thinking."

Although so many teens—and adults!—would have a similar reaction, it, of course, wasn't positive thinking. It was the seemingly upbeat and innocent beginning of a vicious cycle of thought control that would take over Lisa's life and body for the next several years. Millions of you or your loved ones are trapped in that same cycle.

Breaking free of that vicious cycle is the goal. Eating disorders are not only mysterious and difficult to detect, but are often a shameful and carefully guarded secret, making interventions and help even more difficult. In reading Lisa's diary, we are continuously looking for clues to find our way into unlocking the secret places eating disorders hide.

First, it is essential to define eating disorders. Although they seem to center around body image and weight, it is crucial to understand, as this chapter makes clear, that is only a tiny part of the picture. Join Lisa and me in this journey of discovery, as we look for a clearer understanding of the disease in order to begin taking steps toward recovery. Remember, you are not alone.

EATING DISORDERS DEFINED

The media has given much attention to eating disorders, but often without defining them in the first place. Although I will begin by giving some of the technical definitions of eating disorders, that is only a part of the story. Most of the people that eating-disorders professionals see fit loosely into one of these categories, but in reality the categories contain much overlap and the diagnosis is more complicated. For instance, one may have anorexia or bulimia or a combination of the two. Bulimia itself has many faces and may include binging (massive overeating) with purging (vomiting or other means) or exercise bulimia (excessive exercise after binging) as in the case of Lisa (who, in addition, starved herself as a "purge" of the constant binging). It is important to note that like anything else in their lives, for teens, the eating disorder, too, is in a process of transition and change. With adults who have eating disorders, these categories are frequently more defined. Following are some of the more common definitions as described in the *Diagnostic & Statistical Manual of Mental Disorders* (DSM) by the American Psychiatric Association, interspersed with further explanation that should give greater clarity and understanding.

Anorexia Nervosa

Anorexia nervosa is a refusal to maintain body weight at a minimally normal weight for age and height. Less than normal is considered to be less than 85 percent of expected normal body weight. This is usually accompanied by an intense fear of gaining weight. Although these numbers, as shown in standard medical charts, are cited in the DSM, many eating-disorders professionals find it more effective to use a different informal standard. They cite the large variation in body size particularly in adolescents, with many teens being normally very petite and, therefore, smaller than average. A better indicator, therefore, is judging the patient's current weight against her weight at a time when she was eating normally. Particularly in the case of anorexia, even at early onset, the weight drop is usually significant and easily discernable. In Lisa's case, the initial fears were in line with bulimia, although we will see the common "overlap" among eating disorders in the next chapter of the diary when Lisa begins quickly sliding toward anorexia as she graduates high school and readies to enter college.

As the anorectic's weight drops, health is rarely considered. Many anorectics consider themselves in good health despite rapidly escalating health problems. Denial is a key word with the real belief that all that is denied does not exist and they are in complete control of both life and health. One of the most significant early signs of anorexia is the consecutive loss of more than three menstrual periods. This is referred to as amenorrhea. But, again, most anorexics ignore this vital sign.

As we've already read in Lisa's story, detailed records may be kept of food intake, body weight, and measurements. For some, these measurements are taken multiple times per day and are recorded in exact detail. Any variation from the downward curve is cause for alarm. Often this may be accompanied by a distortion in the way the body is seen. Most anorectics actually look in the mirror and, no matter what their real weight, see rolls of fat. As their weight drops even lower, they may be even less able to see the real image. They are not lying about what they see. They really see fat hips, big arms, heavy legs, and a protruding stomach.

What is an equally important indictor of anorexia and other eating disorders is that the sufferer's body shape and weight, at various points, influence the entire perception of the world. We can see this clearly throughout Lisa's diary. If she perceives her weight and body as "good," she feels great. For some the feeling can be something akin to a drug high—especially look for this in the next diary chapter as Lisa finally achieves her "dream" weight. This can create enormous and confusing mood swings. Although all teens experience mood swings, swings associated with eating disorders are much more frequent, more intense, and often more unexpected. In the course of one day, Lisa could feel on top of the world or down in the dumps—always caused by changes in numbers on the scale. As the disease progresses, for many teens, moods may fluctuate with as little as a one-pound weight loss or gain. Sometimes a teen makes a vow to herself to stay off the scale (in much the same way Lisa wrote out contracts with herself), but will get around that by choosing a favorite pair of jeans as a measuring device. Any tightness in the fit of the jeans becomes a call for still greater efforts at weight control. A loose fit (as with Lisa's pants after seeing a nutritionist for what was essentially unneeded weight loss) is cause for euphoria and often a trigger to descend further into the isolation and mind games that are hallmarks of eating disorders.

Bulimia Nervosa

Bulimia nervosa is usually characterized by recurrent episodes of binge eating followed by a purge: often vomiting but also diuretics, laxatives, fasting, or compulsive exercise. Compulsive exercise, often up to 2–3 hours a day, is called exercise bulimia. The DSM defines binge eating as devouring, in an approximate two-hour period, an amount of food that is definitely larger than most people would eat in a similar period of time under similar circumstances. It is also defined as a lack of control over eating during that period.

That's all true, but Lisa's story gives us a much more vivid picture. "The way I eat is definitely weird," she writes at 16. "I'm not always sure why I do it. All I know is, *I must stop* . . . Oh, God, when I think back to every Saturday night for years [babysitting], eating like a pig! The candy, the soda, the cookies, the ice cream, all of the things we never had at home and were encouraged not to eat. How many times did I eat and eat and eat and then run around the house while the kids slept doing push-ups, sit-ups, jumping jacks, anything to erase the Oreos, the Ding Dongs, the cans of Coke, the TV dinners? . . . *I'm fed up with myself.* . . . I hate myself when I do it. I hate myself!"

For many anorectics, denial may remain intact for a long period of time. For many bulimics, like Lisa, the self-hate is not only intense, but often immediate, and efforts are made—like the exercise described or other purging behavior—to immediately undo the damage. As we read Lisa's diary, and as you may have already found out, an important truth becomes apparent—these efforts do not work.

The type of foods consumed by bulimics may vary, but are usually high-calorie or high-carbohydrate choices. It is helpful to talk about this issue, as this is the question most of my clients and those of other eating-disorders specialists pose: "Why do I binge on carbohydrates?" The theory that is most widely accepted as to why most of the binges are carbohydrate based is that the massive binging on such foods (usually high-sugar, carbohydrate-packed foods like candy, cake, cookies, and ice cream) increases tryptophan levels in the brain. Tryptophan is the building block for serotonin, creating a mood of increased well-being and relaxation. Many theorists also say that the body develops a craving for that of which it has been deprived. Most dieters limit carbohydrate intake and thus this becomes what the body craves.

When it comes to bulimia, what has often gotten the most press is the lurid purging option of vomiting. The DSM defines bulimia as including purging behavior that occurs at least three times a week for at least three months. Although valuable for medical diagnosis, this may for all practical purposes be a serious understatement of the facts. Many bulimics purge three times a day or more and, if that purge is vomiting, it may become no longer self-induced, but automatic. The automatic vomiting, with its complete loss of control, is particularly frightening. Although there may be multiple causes for this, what usually occurs is that with repeated vomiting the sphincter muscle becomes incompetent and vomiting is an involuntary reaction. Two other things may also be occurring. The vomiting may also become an adaptive reaction since when the stomach is overfull it begins to hurt. In other cases, the purging is not a regular event and may occur infrequently, centering around weight-loss issues or high periods of stress or transition.

In almost all cases, however, the eating disorder does not even serve as an effective weight-control measure. Therefore, you cannot determine if someone has bulimia based on her weight: She may be slightly underweight, slim, slightly overweight, or more seriously overweight. What is an identifiable symptom, however, is "yo-yo" weight loss and gain. Weight will usually tend to fluctuate with each weight loss followed by a period of weight gain (as we'll see vividly throughout Lisa's diary as she both starts at 15 years old and ends at 22 years old at a perfectly acceptable weight of 120 pounds for her 5'4" frame, but in the middle wildly—even gaining as much as 5 pounds a day— rollercoasters to 145 and every pound in between). Each weight gain will tend to add even more weight than was previously there, in part because the growing body seeks health and normalizing. Later in life, because of a damaged metabolism from the years spent as a bulimic, the body may rebel and refuse to lose weight regardless of eating a healthful amount of calories. What is equally important regarding the yo-yo aspect of weight loss/gain associated with bulimia is that each gain creates an emotional panic, as we see in Lisa's case, and renewed vows and efforts at control drawing the person deeper into the disorder.

Binge Eating Disorder

Binge eating disorder usually (but not always) emerges at a time later than adolescence. It is characterized primarily by periods of impulsive gorging and continuous eating. Many of the same subconscious elements are in play that we've mentioned regarding bulimia and anorexia. There is usually no purging, excessive exercise, laxative or diuretic uses, but there may be various forms of fasting or dieting.

Disordered Eating

Disordered eating is a phrase that unfortunately needed coining because it affects millions of people. It is common, not only among teens and young adults, but people of any age, including senior citizens. Disordered eating refers to a person's attitudes and behaviors focusing on food, exercise, weight, and body shape, causing her to initiate behaviors that may jeopardize relationships, health, happiness, and safety. Initially, it is the preoccupation with how she looks and what she eats. Disordered eating may begin as a means of being more attractive to the opposite sex; athletic weight control; fitting into a prom, wedding, or thirty-year college reunion dress; joining friends in new weight loss methods; or attempting to emulate a favorite model—or even mom, dad or sister. What most people do not realize, as they innocently perform such behaviors, is how quickly disordered eating can spin out of control, take over one's life, or morph into another form of eating disorder, including anorexia or bulimia.

MEDICAL SYMPTOMS

In looking for clues for eating disorders in your own life or that of a loved one, it is important to note the medical symptoms; although, of course, in early adolescence the damage has only just begun. What most teens do not realize is that any emotional or medical symptom is serious and demands attention. Lisa was one of the lucky ones, with few medical symptoms appearing early on. Many people are not as lucky, and you or your loved one may already be seeing some of what I am about to describe. I will briefly discuss the medical problems that begin to emerge at this age, noting that most of these problems are most severe in their future consequences. Please look carefully for these clues as they are frequently overlooked in a standard medical exam. Even in our current sophisticated state of medical practice, eating disorders are frequently misdiagnosed—with the increasing need for the individual or loved one to realize that the medical symptoms they are seeing do indicate an eating disorder and must be addressed.

Some of the anorectic teenagers that enter the office are consuming as few as 400 calories a day. Since 2,000 to 3,000 calories a day is the normal teen intake, they are in a state of starvation. In the simplest terms, this state can be compared to hibernation, with all body functioning slowing down. Normal heart rate is 60 to 80 beats per minute at rest. However, some people with eating disorders have heart rates of 30 to 40 beats per minute. This is very serious, with weakened heart muscles prone to arrhythmia. This creates conditions for heart attack and possible death. Low blood pressure may also cause dizziness and fainting.

Like the missed menstrual periods (more than three in a row) I've already described, changes in body temperature are an early sign of anorexia. Body temperature may consistently fall to about 90 degrees and, in some cases, hands and feet may appear blue. There is a constant feeling of being cold, with the addition of layers of clothing to stay warm. In some cases, lanugo hair may begin to appear on the body, much like the lanugo hair on a baby, as the body attempts to warm itself. This may look like fur and can be frightening.

Gastrointestinal symptoms may include constipation. In bulimics, there is usually a feeling of fullness that occurs after a binge when the stomach is stretched beyond capacity, but may also occur at times when food intake is not the issue and has little to do with real fullness. In anorectics, even the smallest amount of food may cause a feeling of uncomfortable fullness, and a task becomes teaching the person to learn when she is really satisfied. A state of starvation may bring with it abdominal swelling, which may be interpreted as weight gain when in fact it is due to protein deficiency and weight loss. Abdominal pain may be a frequent complaint.

With both anorexia and bulimia, estrogen depletion becomes the norm. What this means is that initially, menstrual periods may stop as the ovaries begin to shut off, creating the potential for problems when the person might want to begin a family. Caught early enough, this is usually reversible. Estrogen is also important for bone strength and, combined with a lack of calcium seen in many eating-disordered patients, creates a major potential problem. Peak bone mass for the rest of one's life is attained during adolescent and young adult years and, although young eating-disordered patients may see no ravages, the effects may be devastating in later years, with a literal crippling of the body in one's thirties or forties. Even earlier than that, we see many stress fractures, particularly in patients, like Lisa, who are exercise bulimics. Osteopenia may occur with teens or young adults, meaning their bone scans will look like those of a seventy year old.

Other medical symptoms also bear mentioning:

■ The use of laxatives, diuretics, and enemas among eating-disordered patients, of course, also pose medical problems. Arrhythmias (discussed earlier) may occur as a result of this abuse. Electrolyte imbalances are frequent and can cause dizziness and fainting.

■ Esophagitis may occur as acid, which is safe in the stomach, pours through the esophagus during vomiting. In severe cases, the esophagus can ulcerate or even split open. Parotid (salivary) glands may also swell as a result of the vomiting, creating pain and a highly visible condition that may look like mumps. A less severe but visible consequence of purging is cuts on the knuckles of the hands used to induce vomiting.

■ All of these conditions are serious, but as we know, the high school years are years of living primarily in the moment. Future medical conditions seem very far away for all teens and the concept of death is often not very real. Teens with eating disorders are no exception to this rule. What my teen clients can relate to is what is immediate and what has to do with how they look. Therefore, the medical avenue that hits closest to home has to do with appearance. With bulimia, teeth are usually affected. Loss of calcium and constant vomiting cause the loss of tooth enamel early on, and weakens the structure of the teeth. The result may be blackened or discolored teeth, serious problems with decay, or teeth falling out, in more severe cases. The hair also suffers. In eating-disordered people, hair may begin to lose color and sheen and in many cases, begin to fall out. Both of these issues cause serious appearance problems. In an age of teeth whitening and hair volumizing, thinking of a smile showing rotting teeth and hair that is limp and thinning and even falling out can be an important visual wake-up call to seek medical and psychological attention.

Biochemical Considerations

An understanding of some of the biochemical brain changes caused by eating disorders and their effect on both thought and mood is rarely written about, and yet I find this information very useful to patients in sorting through their confusion about what is happening to them.

In brief, anorexia produces a state that is similar to starvation, creating an incomplete breakdown of protein in the body and the brain. This leads to the formation of free radicals, which are toxic to the nervous tissue. This toxicity creates problems in thought and mood as well as in memory and intellectual functioning. The incomplete breakdown of sugar also leads to increases in lactic acid, again toxic to the nervous system tissue. In addition, many people with eating disorders are in a hypoglycemic (low blood sugar) state, which may tend to make them lethargic, confused, and irritable with wide mood swings, a quicker anger response, more difficulty in abstract and high-order thinking, and difficulty in determining cause-effect relationships.

In bulimia, an electrolyte imbalance may come on quickly and with little warning. In addition to the deleterious effect of this imbalance on the heart muscles and the weakness, dizziness, and risk of falling that may occur, electrolyte imbalance also affects brain function. Brain functioning in general may slow down with early symptoms including a sense of decreased sharpness, confusion, and numbing. In both cases, depression (as we often see in Lisa's darker diary entries) may be another side effect, with difficulty seeing the future and some sleep disturbance. Within this difficulty seeing the future, everything looks bleak, with no hope for anything good to come or anything to get better, and no ability to see or plan ahead.

A hallmark of an eating disorder is the disconnect between mind and body, and so as the eating disorder progresses, so do the biochemical body changes, creating an even more vicious cycle. You will know you are functioning poorly on all levels, as you become increasingly aware of the perceptual changes, the thought changes, and the mood changes, but you probably will not connect what is going on in your brain with these other feelings. And so until now you may not have thought much about the fact that there was also a brain chemistry effect occurring. As you lose more and more control, you may struggle even harder to regain control. That struggle may involve even greater efforts at restricting your eating and more secretive and sometimes more frequent episodes of binging and purging or exercising—without knowing that part of what is occurring is biochemical and that your actions could be exacerbating the brain chemistry changes.

These biochemical changes are serious, but with an adolescent, these changes are just beginning. The good news—with prompt and proper medical, nutritional, and psychotherapeutic treatment, much is often reversible.

EMOTIONAL AND BEHAVIORAL SYMPTOMS

In addition to the early medical symptoms that may appear for those succumbing to eating disorders, serious emotional and behavioral changes *always* begin to occur. As with many other aspects of eating disorders, these changes can be insidious, not apparent to the affected person or her loved ones until the trap has firmly snapped shut.

If it is during the teen years that an eating disorder takes hold, the often chaotic normal development during this time of life may be difficult to distinguish from behaviors that can be signs of serious problems. Almost all teens, and almost all adults, are concerned about appearance as well as body size and weight, and, therefore, may have moods and behaviors related to these issues that seem a far cry from their previous selves. The biggest question here is where is that thin line and how does it move into what is usually at first disordered eating and then may quickly spiral into a more serious eating disorder? Most therapists see that thin line as defined by frequency, intensity, and duration of symptoms.

How often do you restrict, binge, or purge? Are you preoccupied with thinness, exercise, or body image? Do you think about food most of the time? Are you finding that increasingly this is affecting not only your thoughts, but also your feelings and actions? Are many of your relationships based on body, weight, and food? Are you increasingly focusing on these issues more than most other parts of your world? Is this becoming harder, if not impossible, to control? Are you isolating more in an effort to hide from others? An eating disorder, largely because so much secrecy and denial is involved (Lisa, as we know, confided only to her diary) for years, is often not detected in its early stages. Always remember, though, that early intervention gives us the greatest hope for more rapid and complete recovery.

I will look in a little more detail at that line as I briefly discuss the emotional and behavioral symptoms of eating disorders here, so that you may be able to take the possibly lifesaving step of identifying the disease in yourself or someone you love. Remember, not all of these symptoms apply to everyone, and this should be used as an overall guide to begin to understand what is occurring and to perhaps seek professional help.

Disordered Perceptions

In a person with an eating disorder, perceptual distortions, particularly in the areas of body, weight, and size, may be the first and clearest clue that a problem is developing. During normal adolescence, not only the hormones, but also the body, are in a state of rapid and constant change. Even the bodies of female teens who were firm during childhood begin to fill out and become rounder and more developed in preparation for later child rearing. In a society that at times seems obsessed with thinness, this becomes an issue for many teens. Where is the line? In the development of an early eating disorder, this roundness, particularly in the areas of hips, rounder stomach, and often breasts, is seen as fat—very fat. Often when I meet a client for the first time I see in front of me a beautiful young girl with a developing figure that is to be envied. Inevitably what these same clients see when they look in the mirror is fat. This is what they really perceive on a daily basis, and that image is in sharp contrast to the tall thin supermodel they see in magazines and wish to be. This perception can be painful and overwhelming. They truly hate what they perceive themselves to look like.

Lisa's captured teenaged thoughts broadcast this perfectly: "I am very displeased with myself. I am fat! I am fat! I am fat! I hate myself! Maybe I'm not really fat, but, if that's how I feel, then there's really not much difference. I must change. . . . If I begin now [in March] . . . then by this summer, I should be all set! If I could like myself in a bathing suit that would be real progress! I must begin to feel more secure. I suppose I'm like clay. I can leave myself in a blob [although others saw her as pretty] or mold myself into a work of art."

Knowing about this very real perceptual distortion among those who are developing eating disorders is very important as a clue, especially since what the teen is seeing may not be at all what a loved one is seeing. Any attempt by a loved one to point out the reality will be met by frustration and, in almost all cases, no ability to change the teen's distorted perception. For the eating-disordered person (as this is a hallmark of the disease at all ages), this is not a distorted perception. What she sees in the mirror is her hard, cold, fat, and awful reality. Professional help should be sought.

Disordered Thinking

What will also likely emerge early on are some unusual signs of irrational thinking. The thoughts focus on body image, weight, and food, and are repetitive and obsessive. If you are going through this, you may recognize this as

Lisa did (and will continue to as she also futilely writes about it in future chapters). If it is your loved one, even though she may be secretive about specific eating behavior, her negative thoughts about body image often are broadcast loud and clear. Don't assume this is just normal teen talk, take it as a serious indicator that dangerous behavior may be taking place far from your view.

Catastrophic Thinking

Catastrophic thinking may center not only around food, but also people and situations. Everyone (including the individual) and every situation seems bigger than life. We see this throughout Lisa's diary, when she writes that days are either the "best" or "worst" days of her life and, constantly, how she "must" do this or that, and even signs contracts with herself to fulfill the orders.

Examples of what we are looking for in yourself or others are statements begun by "best," "worst," "always," "never," "must," and "everybody." "Shoulds" (one of Lisa's favorite words) are also present and unfortunately apply to not only what the individual should do, but an increasingly rigid sense of what others around them should do. These "shoulds" can be very tough on loved ones as well as on the person themselves. The one with the eating disorder is not necessarily being judgmental at those points, but rather in a rigid thought pattern and also afraid of the consequences if certain actions do not occur. What I frequently hear from my patients is, "If this doesn't happen [and the "this" may vary from day to day], my life will be over." Some of this thinking is present in all people, especially teens, but again the line crossed depends on frequency, duration, and, most importantly, intensity. For most people with eating disorders, life is always serious with far too little lightness and far too great consequences for almost all of their actions. This is also an important component of the perfectionism and control I will discuss later. One mistake has the ability to lead to dire consequences—to disaster. In some cases, they may have a sense of walking a thin line, a tightrope if you will, with one misstep proving almost fatal.

Our birds-eye exclusive view of examples of this in real words, written as the thoughts occurred, are virtually everywhere in Lisa's diary. These are just a few instances of hundreds peppered throughout:

■ "Well, I ate and I ruined it. Like my life. I'm ruining my life. God help me."

■ "The absolute pits. I reached it today. I was totally unable to cope, to function. I never want to be here again. I can't fit into my TV page work uniform, except squeezed in. . . . I've got to do something, foodwise, besides otherwise. This is a many-faceted nightmare. I'm going to search through all this rubbish, straighten up a bit, and find myself among the ruins."

■ "I do not understand myself to say the least! So cocky, mentally that is. I fell from my tightrope. . . . I know that I hate living in the pits, and I don't ever have to be there. I have control over it. The bottom line is that I feel great when I abstain. Yes, abstain! That Overeaters Anonymous word. Ominous, but true. It's not being perfect or inflexible. It is abstaining from compulsive overeating."

■ "The urge to eat is so strong whenever I feel as though I've overeaten, even by a little. . . . I'm tired of working against myself in the guise of working for myself. . . . It's a circle I get lost in. I get so concerned with staying on that fine line that *is* the circle. If I take a step in, I'll fall in. If I take a step out, I'll fall out."

Black-and-White Thinking

As teens feel more and more out of control regarding their bodies, they increasingly seek to control their thoughts as well as the world around them. This can result in something called black-and-white thinking. Within this, there is a strong sense of the either/or and the good/bad: I am smart or I am stupid. She is a friend or she is an enemy. I can do anything or I can do nothing. He likes me or he hates me, and, most importantly, I love myself or I hate myself, all of which we have already heard Lisa declare a number of times about herself. This black-and-white-thinking is often seen in Lisa's feelings about herself (i.e. I am good; I am bad).

Throughout therapy, one of the tasks is to help the person not only see black and white, but become comfortable with shades of gray. As you will see as you read on, Lisa's boyfriend was always able to do this, but she never adjusted to it and remained tortured by black-and-white thoughts throughout the eighteen-month romantic relationship. In the next diary chapter, too, you will clearly see the flip side of the "love myself/hate myself" part of an eating disorder that you or a loved one also may be experiencing, as Lisa professes her newfound love for herself in entry after entry. That love solely emerged, sadly, because of what she perceived as a major ideal weight loss (in reality less than 10 pounds). Like with so many people with eating disorders, this severe black-and-white thinking will be clear throughout the diary as Lisa boomerangs again and again back to proclaimed self-hatred after not being able to maintain the weight loss.

Magical Thinking and Grandiosity

Magical thinking has to do with a feeling of, "If I will it to be, it will be." In fact, "I will be what I will to be. I will do what I will to do. I want to be. I am," as you will see, becomes a mantra for Lisa. In addition, we might wonder at her daring in sending the ambitious letters to the television networks. It might seem presumptuous for a teen to think about being a TV anchor. But for Lisa, and so many people with eating disorders, this is not at all presumptuous. They have always achieved and often feel that there is nothing they cannot do.

In fact, they are often more surprised than disappointed when what they expect to occur does not happen.

When I asked one of my patients what she dreamed of in the future, she mentioned becoming a supermodel, a TV star, or an Olympic athlete. The problem is compounded by the fact that while these aspirations would seem completely out of line for the average population, many eating-disordered patients (often by high school age) have already achieved goals we might find almost impossible. This adds fuel to the fire of magical thinking—if I will it to be, it will be. She expects, as does Lisa, to be at the top, and, like Lisa, spends much emotional energy comparing herself to others to make sure she remains there. She has been achieving at this level for so long that she has begun to lose awareness of the pressure it takes to maintain this position. She is constantly stressed, but it feels like the norm.

Buffered by strong family ties and constant activity, my patient's less-severe preoccupation with food and weight (disordered eating) in high school spiraled completely out of control in college, when the academic rigors of a top university (nothing else was acceptable) and the resulting inability to remain on top led to a full-blown serious eating disorder. We also clearly see this anxiety later in Lisa as she enters college, finally succumbs to stress, and drops all her classes, shocking her family and friends.

The most serious and dangerous aspect of this grandiosity and magical thinking is its role in the eating disorder itself. At least early on in the disorder there is the feeling of, "I can do anything. I can eat, binge, and purge and it will never affect my health. I have read the medical complications of eating disorders, but they will happen to others, not me. This is just a diet. The hours of exercise I do a day are making me stronger and healthier. I can change what I am doing at any time. I am in control." It is crucial, however, first to recognize magical and grandiose thinking and then to realize it almost always takes professional guidance to change these thought processes.

Mood Swings

If you are already aware you have an eating disorder or if you have identified an eating disorder in a loved one, I don't have to tell you about mood swings. In fact, you are probably an expert. Although in most teens moods vary widely, often even daily or hourly, the mood swings of people of all ages with eating disorders are more severe. As the eating disorder becomes pronounced and the person feels more out of control, the mood swings will increase in intensity, frequency, and duration. If you find this happening to you, you may feel confused and afraid. You will certainly feel out of control. You may even wonder at times if you are going crazy.

These moods are an essential indicator that something is wrong and that you cannot, and do not need to, continue to handle it alone. What is going wrong is that this is no longer normal behavior. You have an eating disorder! Even though it may be difficult for you to know whether the eating disorder has caused these swings or the swings caused the eating disorder, one thing is certain—you will immediately turn to restricting, binging, or purging as a means of numbing the confusion, lack of control, and intensity. And so the cycle is perpetuated. The good news is, as with other symptoms, relief will most likely be in sight if you seek help.

Perfectionism

Eating-disorders professionals are frequently seeing the best and the bright-est—and have to teach them that those qualities, in fact, may have led to their eating disorders. When on the surface everything seems perfect, that probably hints at the heart of the problem itself: perfectionism.

We see this in Lisa from the onset in her first journal entry, as she struggles with concern about grades. "I'm afraid of not doing well. I feel like everyone expects so much of me, including me." That quest for Lisa (and virtually everyone with an eating disorder) extends to a search for the perfect boyfriend, job, and, of course, the perfect body shape. This perfectionism is usually validated by the outside world. In Lisa's case, the high school principal's letter added fuel to the fire by touting, "Another perfect semester. Most people fail to realize the effort that is necessary to achieve this level of scholarship. It takes motivation, dedication and above all hard work." What it took, unfortunately in Lisa's case, is an eating disorder to quell the intense stress and anxiety that is a result of the external, and by teen years the increasingly internal, drive for the perfection that in the real world is never attainable.

What's remarkable in Lisa's diary is that we not only see the perfect veneer that her parents and friends did, principal commented upon, and high school guidance counselor wrote about in his gushing college recommendation letter for her, but how utterly anxious Lisa, the valedictorian/state speech champ/varsity tennis player/newspaper editor-in-chief/girl voted most likely to suc-ceed, felt about all this on the inside.

■ "I eat to escape. Is it possible that I just realized this? Could I be that dense? Didn't I know it all the time? Shove in the food, turn on the TV and tune out; that's the pattern. Now that I'm eighteen, I can write my own excuse notes for school. Escape notes. Do the Winchell's donut run (1 dozen assorted), get the Haagen-Dazs (a pint of mint chocolate), a few cans of Coke and lie down in front of the soap operas in the guest room. Parents at work. Door closed. Just stay outside, Consuela. Don't clean in the guest room today or two days from now or next Tuesday. Lisa is occupying the guest room, Consuela."

■ "Sick and in bed, I think I'll write a few pages to a hypothetical autobio-graphy: Rob Jeffries was the boy voted Most Likely to Succeed in my senior class. . . . The girl voted Most Likely to Succeed should have been Kari Tamner. . . . When I arrived at school on graduation morning, I was shocked to find out that Kari Tamner had not won and that I had. . . . I had gotten out of bed that morning, unlike so many mornings before, only because Dean Belgetti had said that if we didn't come to the final graduation rehearsal we wouldn't graduate. . . . and besides, I was the graduation speaker. On the mornings I didn't go to school, I'd stay home [and eat]. It seemed like I spent half my senior year in this manner. The other half I spent writing my own excuse notes and dropping courses right and left in order to preserve my status as a 4.0 student [and valedictorian]. I was compulsive about those sorts of things, a perfectionist by birth."

At the point they enter therapy, eating-disordered patients usually have no idea that this goal, the goal of perfection, is never possible. It is only later, when trust has been established with the therapist, that the healing tears usually flow and the long hidden doubts, fears, low self-esteem, confusion, and anger are expressed. Thus, the therapeutic process of reconciling the perfect face to the world and the revealing of the true person inside has begun. What is so exciting, is that later in this diary we will see, precisely as it happened— as Lisa goes through therapy with an eating-disorders psychotherapist as well as group therapy—that exact transformation in her, sometimes accompanied by anger, dismay, surprise, and often triumph at the realizations that perfection was the enemy and the prison guard, rather than the goal.

Shame, Guilt, and Secrecy

If you are succumbing to or suffering from an eating disorder, a clear sign is eating in secrecy and feeling extreme guilt and shame afterward. This secrecy is why it is such a treasure to have Lisa's diary as a rare document of an eating disorder. As you are probably all too aware in your own life, people with eating disorders rarely, if ever, share their true feelings or behaviors with anyone. Lisa never told or showed her parents, boyfriends, or friends what was going on in her mind and life. It was a shameful secret with empty food cartons hidden in closets and under beds, until, as you'll see, she later seeks recovery and, hopefully like you, then begins to confide in those important to her—also caught minutes after it happened in her diary.

Control

Nowhere is the issue of control more evident than in eating disorders and how patients deal with weight, food, and body shape. A key similarity among eating-disordered patients is that food, either in terms of restricting or binging and purging, becomes a means of gaining control when the world around them appears to be spinning wildly out of control. We see this as it happened for Lisa—as it does for many females and males, often being the first push into an eating disorder—when she experienced a loss of control in her world as she felt the sting of rejection from a member of the opposite sex. Although, as we read, many boys had been approaching Lisa—and she experienced nothing but accolades from teachers and her principal, all that mattered to her was the actions of this one early crush. Every diary entry before this event was happy, light, and optimistic—and included not a word about weight. Lisa even mentioned that she was cheerfully baking cookies at the moment her crush crushed her. Three months after the incident—the first time she put pen to diary paper again—we see the damage and will continue to see it spiraling wildly for the next three years.

"It's the first time I'm writing without good news," she laments. "I mean I'm not actually depressed, or am I? Nothing seems right. I'm shaky with everything, boys, friends, even family and me. . . . *I will lose the weight and look and feel terrific.*" Lisa never felt she needed to lose weight before (and was, in fact, before that, not overweight at 120 pounds for her 5'4" frame) although there would not be a day again she would feel that way—the loss of control in her world was a key prompt in trying to control her body.

Like in Lisa's case, food issues may begin after even just a slight remark from a member of the opposite sex or a parent. Sometimes, the comment is regarding the person's weight or body shape. In other cases, control regarding the body may emerge with a diet in order to fit into a new pair of jeans or a prom dress. What therapists often see is that the diet may be part of a group effort, a number of teens deciding together to lose weight. What we see far too often are teen bulimia clubs, with binging and purging a means of entry and with a competition regarding who can vomit the most and lose the most weight.

If you recognize this control issue or the others I've talked about so far in yourself or a loved one, that may be an initial sign that help is needed.

SEEKING HELP

It is essential to note here to be careful about the kind of well-meaning help you seek. Some "help" can actually unwittingly become a push further into an eating disorder instead of the other way around. When Lisa's mother noticed that her 16-year-old daughter was becoming preoccupied and upset about her "weight" (although, as discussed, her weight was normal), she asked Lisa if she wanted to visit the nutritionist one of her adult friends was seeing for weight loss. While it's wonderful that Lisa's mother was in tune enough with her to notice this preoccupation, it's too bad that Lisa was not sent instead to an eating-disorders psychotherapist or that the nutritionist did not immediately recognize Lisa's obsession (which, of course, Lisa hid from her) and refer her to one.

Instead, as we see firsthand in Lisa's journal, and many eating-disorders professionals note with their patients, the very plan for healthful eating given to Lisa by the nutritionist (based on the often-used food exchanges developed by the American Diabetes Association) became fuel for the secret obsession, was followed in an unhealthful perfectionist mode by Lisa, and became the model for the obsessive dieting she would follow for years to come—well after the nutritionist bid her goodbye as a "successful" weight-loss case and one of her "best clients ever," when Lisa in just weeks dropped from the 128 pounds she had eaten herself up to down to 116 pounds. (In fact, when Lisa, even lower in weight, came back two years later at age 18 for follow-up help—secretly starving herself, quickly sliding into anorexia, and terrified she was losing even more control of her weight and body—the same popular hospital-based nutritionist commented how great Lisa "looked" and mentioned—as so many misguided people had begun to—"Why in the world does *she* need to be here? She looks fantastic.") This plays up the importance of choosing not only a therapist but all other professionals who are well-versed in eating disorders.

In addition, Overeaters Anonymous played a similar role for Lisa. While relieved for the first time to meet others like herself, Lisa ended up adopting OA's eating philosophy and slogans ("abstaining from compulsive overeating") to an obsessive degree, and used them to continue to imprison herself in her disease for years to come. It is important to realize that Overeaters Anonymous, a very special organization, has proven enormously helpful for so many of my patients, and in some cases has had a lifesaving effect. For Lisa, however, at this point in time, it was not useful.

What is essential, as eventual psychological treatment progresses in an eating-disordered patient, is to unlock the symbolism of what the food behavior really represents. Early on, however, if you notice food control actions in yourself or someone you care about, even if you don't know why they are present, their existence provides the initial and most easily recognizable clues that an eating disorder is developing. As eating-disorders professionals know all too well (and we will be privy to as we continue to read along with Lisa's all-too-common story), it's almost impossible to squelch this kind of thinking and the resulting behaviors on your own. If you or your loved one is informed enough to detect the eating disorder early on, that is the time to ask for help, the kind of invaluable help I will describe to you later in the book, and that you will see being so effective as Lisa fights to first recognize and then break the chains of control that bind her and millions of others.

3. Itsy-Bitsy-Teeny-Weeny Polka-Dot Bikini

18 YEARS OLD

JUNE 20

You are strong.
You will make it.
You can roll with the punches.
You *are* a winner.

I feel so proud. I don't really know why. These things just seem to happen. Even though I have tonsillitis, I know that I've worked hard for this. I tried on my leotards, without tights, and could see no stomach. Wow! Bikini looks nice also. Too much! So much of it is psychological, how you mentally see yourself. I'm walking on a slippery floor and, boy, would it be easy to slip. But I know where I'm going.

Wow.

Weight: 117 pounds

JUNE 24

A milestone. Today, I became an employee, a page, at a television station! Another phase of my life has begun. I knew I could do it, but doing is different from knowing. There is no stopping me now. I think I will make it as far as I want to go. Timing is everything. Wow!

Another thing worth recording: I received a $4,000 college honor scholarship.

JUNE 27

Something is happening to me. It is wonderful, it is dynamic, and, at the same time, it is confusing and scary. I feel different. I think I am emerging as a person, an individual. I don't know exactly what I was before. It's as though I had no personality. I was dull. I was blah. I thought I was grown-up and mature before, but now I feel as though I am really growing.

Although I feel that in essence this has been a day-by-day, very gradual process that I initiated in October, I think three major experiences (events) were catalysts: getting the job, losing weight, and my relationship with Perry. All of these are basically wonderful and, to a large extent, a result of my own personal push. Yet each area creates questions and uncertainty.

When I heard I had gotten the job, I cried. I had done something that deep down I always believed I could. All of a sudden, it seemed my life had been changed (by me). I walked off the street into that television studio, a studio where they said almost 3,000 people a year applied for those page jobs and they only select a few—if any. The future went from being an attainable dream to an attainable reality.

My confidence in myself has made this possible. Where has this confidence come from? It seems relatively new, and yet, I know it's been long in coming. I'll tell you the greatest joy, I like myself, not just one facet, but the whole package. In fact, I love myself, and I feel this is unchangeable. I may go up and down, but I have my own respect now. I think I am beautiful. And although I've written that, I don't feel conceited. This is the way it is. I am a beautiful, pretty, intelligent, talented, motivated, sweet person. I like my body. Although this is not the most important fact, as of today I weigh $115\frac{1}{2}$ pounds. I've worked for it. My long-time weight goal is in sight. I want to protect it once I reach it, so I've decided to go back to the nutritionist I went to two years ago. There I can get a balanced, nutritious maintenance plan.

I love the way I look. I feel I really deserve this. It was not handed to me on a silver platter. Although some say I was always pretty, I don't think I was. (Maybe I was just blinded by self-hatred.) I feel I've molded myself.

I know that looks aren't everything. I thought they were. The personality I never thought I had is emerging. I'm not sure yet what it is. I can be funny and witty. I can be spontaneous. I can be cute. I can be sexy. I can be honest. I can enjoy sex. I can enjoy life. And I can enjoy myself.

I am confused about my relationship with Perry. How do you know if someone is right for you? Through this relationship I have learned to open up and be myself more, yet sometimes I feel like I'm not being myself. He's a very lucky boy to have me.

What makes me such a motivated, goal-oriented person? At eighteen, I feel miles ahead of my peers and friends in this area. I can't sit still. I can't be a camp counselor or a waitress when the world is out there and I am ready to conquer it. What sets me apart? At any rate, I know the things I am doing are making me happy.

All along, I've tried to do the "best" thing, the "right" thing, tried to be the best. Now I just want to be me, no matter what it takes, no matter what I have to do, what images I have to shatter, what approval I must forsake.

I am on the brink of self-discovery and I feel as though a great load has been lifted from my shoulders. I am free to breathe.

JUNE 28

5:19 A.M.

I have accomplished so much regarding my weight and self-image. Looking back, it's taken about a year. Before that everything was overshadowed by self-hatred and insecurity. My first restaurant hostess job last summer made me feel somewhat attractive, yet toward the end I was sneaking rolls, soup, cheesecake, and chocolate syrup (yuk.) At my second hostess job, I also ate bakery items and rolls and bread, and that was as recently as last February.

JUNE 29

This job is going to be *great*. Can you believe it? I got a size-five uniform. I was wearing my size-three purple pants the day I got the job, the day I said to the head of the page staff, "If I don't get this job, I'll go to every studio in Hollywood and knock on doors. And I'll get a job." I couldn't believe the things I said. It was like I caught fire the minute the guard said they were interviewing for pages. I knew if there were openings I could get a job. And I did. Last interview out of the whole group she had been interviewing for months and first hired the very next day. Wheee!

This job is going to be great. A cameraman already told me I was beautiful, looked like a beautiful Spanish senorita, and asked me to go sailing (which I won't).

But it is a lot more than this attention. Where was I today? On the set of a national talk show having a superstar guest tell me, "Just keep smiling and you'll make it," as he walked out onto national television.

I am here. I made it in. I am surrounded by "the beautiful people," and, by some miracle, I have become one of them.

JULY 2

Things seem to be going very well now. Nevertheless, the past casts a shadow I can't ignore. I have a disease. I am a compulsive overeater.

Although the symptoms, outer flab and inner insecurity, may have disappeared, the germ of the disease remains. Just as a diabetic must take his daily doses of insulin, I must take my daily doses of positive thinking.

I am me and that is good enough. It never was before. Who am I? That is a question that I am answering and will continue to answer every day for the rest of my life. Sometimes my findings will be pleasing, sometimes not. But I will be accepting. I accept myself.

I have confidence and strength. I am only beginning to tap these resources. By losing weight I have conquered my own inner demon. Consequently I will never be defeated by life.

I can't say that I am used to myself yet. I can't say that I truly know myself yet. But day by day I come face to face with a welcome stranger and a new-found friend.

JULY 4

An analogy came to mind today. My room reflects me, not only the possessions, but the manner in which it is kept. To the eyes of others, it is always perfect. If it is not up to par, no one sees it. Period. Most of the time it is in a state of mess, clutter, and confusion. I cannot seem to keep it up.

I used to project that same kind of "neat" image to the world. Every hair had its place, and every hair in its place. Smile, smile, smile. Don't let anyone see you unless you look perfect. But what was underneath that false exterior? A mess. Anger, self-hatred, self-punishment, and denial. Clutter.

Luckily, or purposely, I am changing. Letting my hair down, or more appropriately, in my case, putting it up. Letting loose and letting go. It's hard not being so hard on myself.

I am less than perfect. It's also hard to admit, but now I'm not sure what I'm striving for. Before, it was perfection pure and simple (or, I should say, polluted and difficult—impossible). What I want now is to be the best me I can be. How do I know when I get there?

JULY 6

The ultimate test: Can I really go to a roller-skating rink wearing a skin-tight rainbow tank top?

(Scratch that! We couldn't go.)

I look in the mirror and I like what I see. In the past, this would have seemed like a miracle. Now at times I'm even blasé. I realize, however, that I could never really be blasé about it. I worked too hard. This *is* a tremendous (or rather "trim"-endous) accomplishment.

I look inward, and I like what I am beginning to sense, an assertiveness. Passiveness is passé. Shyness is turning to sensitivity. As my shell grows tougher—I can take almost anything now—I grow softer. My growth actually has been phenomenal. I realize now that I have never really known myself. It was as if I had hated a stranger, someone I had never taken the time or courage to get to know.

Well, now it is a totally different ball game. I am continually hitting singles, doubles, triples, and even home runs. I won't forget my past strike record, however. While I appreciate the cheers from the crowd, they are not essential. My own congratulations mean more than all the applause in the world.

This, I think, is a phase. I am discovering my identity. When I grow to know myself more fully I will be comfortable and content.

I am special. I may be good. I may be bad. But I am special. Deep inside I know that I will make it in every way.

JULY 7

My life is consistently wonderful. This is not to say that everything is coming up roses. I am the rose. It may be raining upon me. The ground around me may turn to mud. I may be left to grow alone, yet, I, myself, remain calm, peaceful, strong, stable, and subtly beautiful.

I am full of pride. I have done a great thing by losing weight and continuing to do so. I am only beginning. Life holds beautiful things in store for me, because that's what *I* hold in store for life!

JULY 8

Bust: 36"   Abdomen: 32"!
Thigh: 20"!   Lower leg: $12\frac{1}{2}$"
Waist: 25"!   Calf: $7\frac{1}{2}$"
Hips: 35"   Upper arm: 10"!

JULY 8

I have come full circle. Mine is a life worth living. I have achieved. I have accomplished. I have become. I have arrived.

Life is no longer torment. Life is no longer misery. Life is no longer punishment. Life is no longer repression, denial, self-hatred, or insecurity.

Life is mine. Life is challenging. Life is adventure. Life is acceptance. Life is calm, serene, and peaceful. Life is courage, strength, and confidence. Life is joy beyond ecstasy. Life is love, simple in its complex intricacies. Life is living. I have grown up. I have taken the reins of my life in my own hands. I grabbed control.

Day by day, moment by moment, setback by setback, goal by goal, pound by pound, I created the love I now feel for myself. Without being able to foresee the future, I believed in myself. I was not my ideal person or weight, yet I sensed my potential and never gave up on the toughest enigma, myself.

So much of the growth was subconscious. It took place, oh so gradually, beneath the surface. Before, I had only tried to alter, repair, and cleanse that surface, never even guessing at the special fountain that lay deep within.

I am only beginning to tap that fountain.

JULY 15

There is nothing wrong with the way I am eating or not eating. Everyone keeps saying I should eat more. I tell them I am not hungry.

I am finally 113 pounds. I am finally a size three. I bring my can of chocolate liquid protein that I stock up on from the supermarket to work everyday, and, when I reapply my make-up on my break, I drink it. I have two or three more cans a day. I'll start eating again soon. Sometimes I eat a little, I've been not eating for only about a month. I'm really not that hungry anymore.

I am thin. I am happy. And that's all that matters for now.

JULY 23

Well, well, well, life is always changing, isn't it? What I am about to record is by no means a fact. It is just a reaction, an impression, that I have as of today.

I think I may have put it in perspective (at least mentally). It was a high school relationship. We are better friends now than ever. We have a beautiful friendship. I think we were both so scared at the newness before that we couldn't *really* get to know each other. We were always concerned with such trivial, surface things. Now it's easier to talk, really talk.

It is probably time to move on. Something has changed. The future. Before I hoped Perry would be a big part of it. Now, I don't think he will. Although I am by no means sure.

It was nice, and a growing experience.

But there's a whole world out there. It would be naive and foolish to believe that there is only one person who can make you happy.

JULY 24

Things have truly fallen into place. I am whole, and I am beautiful. Today, Greg Butler, a terrific person, became interested in me. What will happen I am not sure. But he is extraordinary and extraordinarily good (great) looking.

We have a date for tomorrow night.

My life is looking up.

JULY 25

Another momentous first date. Where it will lead, who knows? What's more important is the here and now. Jumping from Perry to Greg is like jumping from one cutie-pie to another. I can't believe we've both been working as pages at the television studio for over a month and had never even met before. What a kiss!

JULY 27

Surprise after pleasant surprise. I can't believe he called me so quickly, the minute I got home from my graduation present gift with Cheri to San Diego, even though it was so late. I think I am becoming involved (I am) with a very special (spectacular and unique) person. I am excited, and yet I am calm (and confident and competent). To say Greg is gorgeous is superficial. That's what his modeling and acting are for. However, there is so much more to him than that.

True, we've only known each other a short while, yet it is very comfortable. This is another measure-meter of my progress. I am different. I am fulfilling my potential. As he quite appropriately put it, "Sweet dreams."

JULY 28

2:14 A.M.

Well, Greg certainly is unique. I've never met anyone like him. Wow, I'm not sure what I think yet. I'll have to get to know him better.

I know, though, that when we have these marathon late-night phone conversations, I am entranced. He does impressions. He talks to me like Jack Nicholson. But who needs anyone else? I am charmed. He is charming. At twenty, the oldest person I've been out with. He is so smooth; there's something very special there. He's on fire, like many of the pages, but more so. He is not just a pretty, vacant Bel Aire boy. True, he's pretty. And he definitely comes from the "right side of the tracks." But he has the charisma and energy that would take him to the top of the business world regardless of where on the ladder he started.

This is a time in my life I will always remember. Everything should not be taken so seriously.

JULY 28

Bust: 35"!	Thigh: 19"!
Waist: 24"!	Lower leg: $11\frac{1}{2}$"
Hips: 32"!	Calf: 8"
Abdomen: $29\frac{1}{2}$"!	Upper arm: 10"

AUGUST 5

I am a different person. Both inside and out. I really haven't been aware of the full extent of my change. I look different. I am a size three as opposed to a size seven or nine. Consequently, my face and body are not the ones I was used to seeing (if I really did see).

As for my personality, it hasn't changed, it's emerged (because it wasn't there before). I *am* a different person.

I remember reading about how a former fatty must mourn for her "fat self," someone she has had such an intensive love-hate relationship with for so long. I also remember thinking that this did not apply to me. That was then; this is now. I believe I am grieving. It has begun to hit me that the old me is gone, really gone. I don't know where she is. She must be dead. A big part of me has died. Although, for the most part, I didn't like this person, I cared about her.

Not liking yourself is misery, but it becomes routine and almost comfortable. Now knowing yourself, however, is scary as hell. I'm terrified and yet confident that in time I will come to know the mysterious, compelling stranger who stares at me from the other side of the mirror.

AUGUST 7

3:00 A.M.

Putting things in their proper perspective is not an easy task. For example, I am not sure what I look like. Sometimes I see one thing (a fat, ugly person), sometimes another (a thin, pretty person). What is real? I am not sure. What do others see?

Everything is confusing. But I will keep hanging on, taking one day at a time and enjoying life.

I may be falling for Greg, a total cutie-pie. That, too, I will take as it comes.

AUGUST 9

Redirect that anger and reassess it. Greg didn't mean to upset you by not going with you to the party. Assess what's important, and then go for it. Don't waste time being mad or eating over being mad. Don't give up, no matter what.

Don't compromise and don't settle.

You can be the weight you want to be.

Do it. Your way.

AUGUST 10

Another crossroad along the path of self-discovery: I find that I can't just settle for being "thin" or "trim" or "fit" or "in good shape."

What is it, then, that I want, and is it realistic? Am I setting myself up for failure and self-defeat? I want to be a knock out! I want to be in great shape. I want to have a terrific figure. I want to look fantastic (and feel that way, too).

Truthfully, I am already pretty, slim, and attractive. I have a very good figure. And my self-image has greatly improved. But, damn it, I am not going to stop short of my goal again. I will not sell myself short.

My goal is realistic because I am not aiming for perfection. Perfection has been a major flaw in my character. No more. I am human. I do make mistakes. But, I do think I can be better (not perfect, just better). What, in all honesty, I want is to be the very best I can be. Anything less is a cop-out.

I feel my potential is immense. Why stop at A– when you have A+ potential?

P.S. In order to squelch all fears of crazed dieting (i.e., anorexia), I will set a conscious weight that I will not go under (without serious consideration): 103 pounds.

AUGUST 12

Another journey begins.
Seek and you shall find: 103 pounds.

AUGUST 17

Boy, has my life changed. Me. Me has changed.

Perry. I love him. I do. I guess I jumped the gun when I thought our relationship was over. I don't know if I'm "in love" with him or if I just plain love him. We are so special, together and apart. We are and have been good for each other. After not seeing each other, when he kissed me and told me I looked beautiful, it felt right. (I knew I looked beautiful. After all, I was wearing a gorgeous satin magenta size-five dress!)

So it turned out for the best, after all, that Greg couldn't go to Lynne's birthday party with me. I was mad, since she's my best friend and I wanted him to meet her. If he had come, though, I might never have re-discovered Perry. I decided that Perry is a beautiful boy who will someday be a beautiful man, who I may or may not have all of, but who I nevertheless will always remember.

AUGUST 18

First, I want to record Greg, my "other boyfriend" for posterity. Very nice. He's extremely good-looking. He's got "it," the "glow," which, incidentally, I've decided Perry has acquired, too, just as I have. Blond (white blond), straight, nicely cut hair. Big light blue eyes. Great smile. Charm. Nice nose. Six foot two inches. Very slim, but looks excellent in clothes and has excellent taste. He's a unique person who's beginning to grow on me. I like him. But I still have deep, special feelings for Perry. I don't know Greg well enough to make any judgments, but I'm glad he's around.

What am I doing? Foodmania has entered the picture again. Although there is a difference, I'm not guilt ridden. (Not that I'm thrilled.) I think I do it to deal with frustration, anger, fear of sexuality, anxiety over moving out and starting a new life in college. Okay, so you know partly why you do it, so *why* do it?

Lisa, you know what you have to do, you have to cut this shit out for good, you have to reach your ideal dream weight. You're so close. And you, Lisa, can do anything. You are you, and that ain't chopped liver!

Why pull yourself down like today? Why couldn't you have just gone to Pierre's going away party? You swam. You sat by the pool in your skimpy bathing suit, and you knew you looked good. Yes, it was a lot different than parties of years before. Yes, you felt like a different person. Yes, it was weird. So Greg couldn't go, couldn't sit next to you at Pierre's beautiful Beverly Hills pool and spa. What's the big deal? These people are all wonderful and all your new, but already good, friends from the page staff. Why did you have to stop at that supermarket on the way? No, two candy bars might not have seemed like a big binge before, but now it's huge. And on the way home? A pint of ice cream is right back down your old path. Things were supposed to be different now. At 112 pounds things are supposed to be different.

Something just hit me. I want to stop. For good. What is more important than anything in my life is to be an abstaining compulsive eater and to be able to eat, rather than just drinking liquid protein, and still be abstaining. (The restricting to liquid protein seems to be losing its charm, judging by today.) This is the only thing that can separate the future from the past, tomorrow from today.

It is the most important thing in my life.

I will do it because I have to.

I love me.

AUGUST 21

I want to have no stomach.
I want a little butt.
I want skinny fingers.
I want a thin face.
I want firm boobs.
I want a *small* waist.
In other words—*I want it all.*
GO FOR IT!!!
Current Weight: 115 pounds

AUGUST 26

What is happening? Am I losing sight of reality?

Stop fooling yourself.

Do you want to throw away your life? Stick a knife in your back? Give up freedom for slavery? It *is* your choice.

Is it finally hitting you? Food in excess is *poison.* It is.

A bag of chocolate chips. A whole bag of marshmallows. Come on! This is a problem that is not going to go away. Go ahead, cry. But you can *do* something.

You can be as strong as you can be, strong enough to forgive, not forget.

This condition is controllable. So learn how to control it.

In this case, the end (weight loss) does *not* justify the means (total starvation.) You thought it did.

Now you know a little better.

And you're learning every single minute.

AUGUST 31

I feel so gorgeous! Maybe I have only lost three pounds, but thin really is just as much a state of the mind as of the body. It is, indeed, a state that must be fought for, protected, and appreciated, whether consciously or unconsciously, every day of your life.

Taking off excess weight is no easy task. However, the true test, the real tough stuff, is keeping off the weight, and the negative self-image, permanently.

Feeling great takes work. Feeling lousy comes naturally; you don't have to work at it.

I'd rather work for the first option, and it *is* an option, a choice. Life is choices.

Positive thinking is *the* most valuable tool in a valuable life. A helpful motto for me has been:

I will be what I will to be.

I will do what I will to do.

I want to be!

I am.

I love life.

SEPTEMBER 1

Keeping it off is the hard part.

I didn't compulsively overeat.

Eating is not compulsively overeating.

I *am* beautiful.

SEPTEMBER 2

I am a product of myself.

I am not a product of chance.

I am not a product of nature.

I am my own artist, creator, designer.

4. Overwhelmed

18 YEARS OLD

A new phase. Another one. College. Here I sit in my dorm room. Solid impressions have not yet set in. It is new and exciting. One interesting note: when asked to list our priorities, others wrote, get good grades. For me there was no question, be happy.

Everything is an outgrowth of that state of mind. Other things fall into place. Well, I've changed. I do feel calm and peaceful.

Like, I can take it.

Today, I became a college student. But, oh, I have become so much more than that. I am finally thin. The calmness and serenity that come from that fact are a subtle backdrop to life now. The realization that "I can" has blended in. Happiness is only a part of it. Contentment is the key word. That is more inclusive. It's not like everything is wonderful all the time, but life, itself, is wonderful. It's true you may have to dig through tons of dirt to find a few diamonds, but that makes the digging worthwhile and gives it purpose, meaning, and significance.

I will be what I will to be.
I will do what I will to do.
I want to be.
I am.

I hope my electric wok isn't stinking up the dorm room, but I can't eat that dorm food. Meal ticket, meal ticket, go to waste. Tough luck. I cried to my mom when I asked her to bring my wok and told her I couldn't use my meal ticket except for cereal for breakfast. I felt so bad that I was wasting their money—so much of it is being spent here—but she said, "Don't worry about it. Just be happy." The point is, though, if sometimes I'm going to eat normally and sometimes drink my liquid protein (pretty expensive for me), then dinners have to be light (chicken, vegetables, etc.). I'll cook them in my wok and wash it out in the bathroom.

Mashed potatoes, bread, cake, cookies: Forget it. I gained five pounds in the first week and a half. There's no way that's going to happen to me.

Not *me*. Not the girl who has suddenly become a potential campus star. I mean I saw it coming this summer with the reaction I got at my job, but this is incredible.

Nice-looking guys asking me to dance. A lot of guys. Everywhere I go I'm getting asked out. This is amazing. A dream.

And there's still Perry and Greg. And me, in my little tight tank top, a tank top girl finally, charming the pants off everybody.

Just hold on and enjoy the ride.

SEPTEMBER 27

". . . Despite the fact that I am meeting many new people every day, I find that I miss you very much. I do hope to see you again soon, or at the very least continue a correspondence if you do not wish to go out anymore, but I hope you do."

Love,
Perry

SEPTEMBER 30

Love is confusing. I really don't understand the way I've been feeling. I was so depressed. I kept thinking about Perry, about us. I was hurt and upset that he didn't even call, let alone see me, before I moved into the dorm. Then, when I got his letter I was ecstatic. What causes these intense feelings? Is it love? Really love? I know I love him. But is it the *real* thing? Is it important that I know? I want to see him and be with him. I miss him.

OCTOBER 3

Bike, take me through this pretty campus. I am so glad that I brought my bike. Five miles a day, everyday, should do it. Keep me fit. After classes on weekdays make myself do it. On the mornings before work make myself. Weekends get up and do it.

I can think. I can feel bad thoughts leave me. They fly out in the wind. My face is flushed. My breath hard. I breathe in life, a life that is and will be special.

OCTOBER 5

God damn it. What the hell do you think you're doing?

May I have change for a dollar? And another dollar and another? Some change will buy you a Snickers. A little more change, a bag of M&M's. A bit more, some peanut butter cups. All from an anonymous machine. No one to see you turn red. No one, not even a cashier, to know what you're doing.

You had it made, Miss. Dance, dance, dance. Smile, smile, smile. They see you and they like what they see.

So why again? Why, why, why? It's not the amount anymore. Three bars is not as outrageous as the whole bags of your yesteryears. That's the point: There's no choice. You don't want to, but you do. That's no choice.

Go ahead, be scared. You should be, Beauty.

OCTOBER 7

I don't want to be misleading. I mean, I don't want to look back on this next year and read about how miserable my life was. Because it's not. Overall, I have been feeling and looking exceptionally well. Almost every day I reflect on the goodness and calmness of my life. I have direction. My page job is wonderful. Life, itself, is wonderful, I think.

I have never been this popular. I could never even have imagined being this popular.

Today, however, and many other times, I feel quite mixed-up. Honestly, *I have come so far.* Just a year ago I had no conception of who I was or what I was capable of. Now I am in college, and I am adjusting. Yet things are missing. Or rather, I am missing home, Perry, etc. I just don't know how I feel. I feel different. As if I am like no one else.

Do I have a lifelong problem with eating? Somehow, I feel the answer is yes. Am I being too subconsciously stringent? What should I do? I love myself and I want to help myself.

OCTOBER 9

I'm going to take a little trip Friday, Saturday, and Sunday. Self-directed. Not a lifetime, just three inner-directed days to get a push. I will not worry about other people. Just me. Just minimal food and maximum exercise. A time to recap and recoup. Walk, jump, dance, run . . . a minute at a time.
Destination: Monday morning.

OCTOBER 27

If this sounds jumbled it's because that's how my thoughts are. Well, I'm changing again, physically, and, I suppose, mentally and emotionally, too. I've decided that there is more to being thin than being thin. Being thin does not mean being happy, feeling good or even, necessarily, looking good. It takes more. I think for me, it takes eating a balanced diet (not just refraining from binging). Plus it takes a fitness program and lots of positive thinking.

My life is so interesting and Perry is the most pleasing part. I guess there's no real way to judge what a true everlasting love is. All I know is that for now I am in love. There really is little question left in my mind.

And he loves me.

There are other boys and men and boys and men and boys. I'm used to it now. Me, a heartbreaker, cheerleader, homecoming queen type? That's how people see me.

I seem to be constantly changing. I try to help myself and understand myself in whatever ways I can.

OCTOBER 30

Perry,

You are a wonderful person.
Whether you realize it or not,
I realize it.
Don't think you are mixed-up. Everyone is confused.
Everyone.
Your mother was right about being able to live.
Let yourself.
Know that nothing you could ever, ever do to me could be wrong.
Don't twist what happens in your mind. It's natural and normal.
Just let it happen.
Then let it be.
Know yourself well enough to know what you want.
Go for it, with no regrets, no guilt.
You are capable of anything.

Lisa

OCTOBER 31

I can't take this anymore. Up. Down. Up. Down. Is there no in-between? Where am I?

I am in classes. They are hard (biology, freshman composition, communications, critical graduate cinema), but I am working hard and doing pretty well. Now my cinema professor is telling us we must read German articles (in German!) for our mid-term. Why in hell did I take a graduate cinema course? I didn't know when I enrolled that it was a graduate course, and the description sounded easy. And now the bombs are dropping, and so am I.

I know one thing, with Gary and Rob coming over to study biology (Gary on Tuesdays, Rob on Thursdays), I have changed. Gary is on the USC baseball team. Rob is Rob, and that's saying a lot. Ironically, that's the same Rob who I was thrilled to invite to my sweet sixteen party. The same Rob who was the most popular boy—Homecoming King, star athlete, star student at my high school. We two, both named "Most Likely to Succeed," were the only students ever from our new high school to go to USC. And now, he's my study partner in my dorm room. Sitting a breath away. Unreal. We're all smart here and that doesn't even matter anymore.

The point is, I don't understand myself anymore. I finally thought I had everything that I wanted and I still eat. Not as much and not as often, but they're still binges and I still hate myself when I do it. Why screw up such a wonderful (?) life?

NOVEMBER 1

"Mom, oh, Mom, please help me." That's what I said today. Finally, I had to tell someone I need help. I can't take it anymore.

I was hysterical in the phone booth. "Mom, I think I heard it's bulimia, but I don't throw up, so I don't know what exactly it is. But there is something wrong with me. I gorge and starve; gorge and starve and then force myself to try and exercise all the calories off my body. I should not be like this. I am ruining my life. I'd rather leave school and fix myself. I can't go on like this. Will you call your doctor and find me a doctor, anyone, to help me?"

I am coming home, Mom. Welcome me back to your arms because I can't take it.

P.S. Don't tell Dad until we have to pay somebody. We'll tell him I'm switching schools next semester because I don't like it here. I'll live at home and go someplace cheaper.

NOVEMBER 2

I am calmer now.

Tomorrow will be a turning point whether I decide to leave school or stay. Live, love, laugh, and learn. I am trying to help myself. Why should I make my life miserable by gorging and playing cruel tricks on myself? I told myself yesterday, "If you go out and eat those candy bars while you should be studying for your communications test, you leave the dorm for home immediately. Consequently, you will not study, you will miss a mid-term and you will never be able to come back to school again."

I ate. I went home last night. I missed the mid-term today.

I am a terrific person. Why am I afraid of that terrificness? Why won't I let myself enjoy the benefits of my healthy, trim, serene, beautiful existence?

NOVEMBER 3

Read between the lines of your life.

You will be amazed at the incongruity.
That which is beneath the surface, is the surface.
Yet it is hidden, repressed.
The spaces between the lines reveal more than the lines themselves.
What are the lines except empty words filling an empty page?
It is what goes on between those lines that is the true essence of your life.

NOVEMBER 5

FOOD

Breakfast:
1 slice wheat bread
1 tbsp. peanut butter
1 cup non-fat milk
$\frac{1}{2}$ medium apple

Lunch:
2 slices wheat bread
2 oz. roast beef
1 cup fruit salad
diet dressing

Later:
1 large package banana chips
2 Snickers bars
2 Baby Ruth bars
1 large Chunky bar

I've got to cut this out. This is so stupid.

EXERCISE:

Stairs:
up 3 times
down 3 times
1 long walk
150 hula hoops

NOVEMBER 6

The minute I start feeling really good, it happens again. I eat and eat and eat to erase the good feeling.

What's wrong? Why won't I let myself be?

NOVEMBER 8

5:36 P.M.
One minute,
    you wake up
and realize,
    it's time
to take responsibility
    for your life.

Getting Thin
Is Not the Answer

We live in a world that is obsessed with thinness. Spurred by media hype and airbrushed pictures of astonishingly thin models, movie, and TV idols, children as young as five are already acutely aware of weight. Years ago, I watched through a one-way mirror my daughter's nursery school classmates and heard the words, "We are not going to Jill's birthday party. She's too fat!" I remember being both angry and shocked. I remain angry. I am no longer shocked. At age five, Jill learned a painful lesson about weight. Fat was not acceptable, and she was already being excluded.

According to current statistics, 42 percent of the girls in grades 1–3 want to be thinner. By age 10, 81 percent are afraid of being fat. In the 9–11 age range, 82 percent have family members who are sometimes, or very often, on diets, and 51 percent of the 9–11 year olds report feeling "better" by dieting. By college, 91 percent have attempted to control their weight by dieting. Although in somewhat different form, boys are, of course, part of the picture, too, with statistics rapidly increasing each year of those who are weight and body concerned and those with eating disorders. An estimated 35 percent of "normal" dieters progress to pathological dieting, and 20–25 percent progress to partial- or full-symptom eating disorders.

And so thinness becomes their utmost goal, one that they believe will solve all of their problems. The only problem is that it is all an illusion, an illusion that, as in Lisa's case and millions of others, becomes a desperate trap—a trap that's both emotional and physical. A trap that will remain until you better understand what is really happening and find the courage and strength to reach out for help.

But, for now, Lisa, like perhaps yourself or your loved one, is stuck, stuck in the mind game that thinness is everything. You've seen her euphoria from losing less than ten pounds, and you've already seen the beginning of a breakdown when that euphoria begins to wear off and she reluctantly starts to meagerly eat again, rather than starve herself. It would be helpful to take a look at how these thought processes work. That will be your first step in breaking free from them.

WHY ME? WHY NOW?

If we have had strong cues since we were small children to desire thinness, why does an eating disorder sometimes not evolve until the teen years, college, young adulthood, or even later? Let's begin by exploring that issue.

The years between the ages of 12 and 21 are particularly high risk for the development of an eating disorder. We begin with Lisa in high school—a time when so many of my patients enter treatment. In today's world the high school years are plain and simply tough. We live in a world of innumerable choices about every area of life including activities, friends, interests, and more significantly career choices, sexuality, alcohol, and drugs. Pressure is everywhere; at the same time, life around us is rapidly changing. Not only outside, but also inside, our bodies are changing, and at times the whole world may seem confusing, unpredictable, and out of control. It is against this background that eating disorders emerge. However, my patients who come to me during their teen years are the lucky ones—they have caught their disease at the earliest stage.

How do these eating disorders begin? For a limited few, their eating disorder comes as a result of a serious or traumatic event. But, for most, the eating disorder creeps up slowly and insidiously, in time controlling all thoughts and actions. That is exactly what happened to Lisa. In the early chapters, we see the slow emergence of her preoccupation with body size, increasing measuring and charting of food and body measurements, and brief glimpses into the extent of her binge eating and patterns of secrecy. Excessive exercise patterns have also begun to emerge. It is difficult to say exactly when the line is crossed, but we are made aware of a number of pivotal moments. For one, at the end of her senior year in high school, Lisa becomes ill with pink eye and tonsillitis. Drugged and dozing for days, she was unable to eat. The result was a rapid weight loss and numbers on the scale she had never before been able to achieve (even though it was less than a ten-pound loss!) Lisa saw this fluke as a miracle. She could lose all of the weight that she wanted, and the way to do it was purely and simply to stop eating and drink only the liquid protein shakes she stocked up on.

For Lisa, this rapid weight loss, this "success," served as a trigger. For so many of my patients, this same trigger-effect occurs. They have a sudden drop in weight due to an illness, or they may be preparing for a special event, for instance, a period of restriction to fit into a prom dress or to " look great" for another special occasion. The trigger may be the "tutoring" from a good friend in the benefits of bulimia, a weight-loss "competition" among peers (we're all dieting together), or a period of restricting to impress a new guy. The trigger may be a seemingly simple, innocent remark by a boyfriend or parent, as were some additional pivotal moments for Lisa. It may also be a very specific remark by a coach, ballet teacher, or other valued adult about additional weight loss contributing to looking better or better performance. In many cases, there is a trigger. In all cases, the weight loss is rapid and the numbers on the scale reach unprecedented proportions.

The result of this weight loss is heady. Some of my patients describe it like the intoxicating effects of a first drink or a drug-related high. Lisa's euphoric writing certainly reflects it. This high begins to cloud thinking and perception and create distortions. Black-and-white thinking that I described earlier begins to emerge, and with it a heightened sense of grandiosity. Everything is beautiful and great and wonderful. Even the loss of a few pounds becomes intoxicating. A gain of any amount really does feel devastating. In most cases, the result is the same as Lisa's—to want more, not only of the weight loss, but, more importantly, also the top-of-the-world feelings associated with it. Without knowing it, almost innocently, you have begun the addiction. The illness has taken hold and you have crossed the very thin line entering the road to destruction.

TRANSITIONS

The period of years between the ages of 17 and 21 is also a period of tremendous transitions. This adds greatly to the risk of either developing or intensifying an eating disorder. We'll look a little more closely at some of these transitions, particularly in the area of identity, and what to expect.

Identity Transitions

The years following high school can be an exciting time. For most people, either going away to college or simply leaving home means a new start. That may mean leaving behind all that they have ever known including friends, family, home, and community. They are moving to a new place where no one knows anything about them. For many, this is seen as a time to, in effect, reinvent themselves. It is a second chance to be the person they have always wanted to be. Lisa writes: "I am a different person both inside and out. I really haven't been aware of the full extent of the change." Most of my eating-disordered clients were stars in high school, again the brightest and the best, but they were also perfectionists who never saw themselves as quite good enough. They see the summer before high school as a chance to prepare for a new beginning. Like Lisa, they feel (often erroneously) that they have been an A- and are no longer satisfied with being an A-. They begin to prepare for a college career that is nothing short of A+. They firmly believe that the A+ centers in part on the perfect body.

"I look different." Lisa writes. "I am size three as opposed to size seven or nine. Consequently, my face and body are not the ones I was used to seeing (if I really did see). As for my personality, it hasn't changed, it's emerged (because it wasn't there before.) I am a different person."

The key concepts are, "if I really did see" and "because it wasn't there before." Despite all of her wonderful successes, Lisa had never developed a strong sense of internal identity. What has begun is a not-uncommon distortion of past reality. Lisa sees herself, the star of so many things in high school, as having been nothing. She begins to base the sense of who she is on her body. She remembers not who she was, but how she looked. She negates the past attraction of high school boys and sees her slightly heavier high school body as both unacceptable and belonging to a different person. What she sees as a change in her personality has purely and simply to do with a radical change in her body. Slowly but surely, Lisa's concept of herself and her concept (at times distorted) of her body become one and the same. She is her body.

For many others, the scenario is a little different. But regardless of the individual situation, beginning again can be frightening. There are not only new possibilities but also new questions. Who are my friends? Where do I fit in? How do I get to know my new surroundings? Will I date, have a boyfriend, find love, establish a lasting relationship? How can I do all the work? Will I succeed? Will I excel? Will I stand out in the crowd? Will I even be able to hold my own? I have always been known and stood out. Now, I feel invisible. I am supposed to be a great student and have a great social life, how can I do it all? I CAN DO IT ALL. Everyone I know has such high expectations for me. I have such high expectations for myself. The demands are enormous. The demands are conflicting. Everyone tells me this should be the best time of my life. HELP ME!

In college even more than in high school, the stakes in the positive answers to these extremely stressful questions are enormous. As you try to answer these questions, you find yourself strangely alone, having left behind people, places, and past victories that have served as anchors and held you together. The past identity that you have so carefully built is gone. The thought of being on your own and having to be independent can be very frightening despite the false bravado that you, like Lisa, will surely attempt to show. Lisa writes: "Not liking yourself is misery, but it becomes routine and almost comfortable. Not knowing yourself, however, is scary as hell. I'm terrified and yet confident that in time I will come to know the mysterious, compelling stranger that stares at me from the other side of the mirror."

All previous anchors are also gone leaving not only anxiety, but also a gaping hole. That hole cries out to be filled and it quickly becomes apparent that a way of filling the hole is with food, often-large quantities of food. In addition, large quantities of high-sugar and carbohydrate-laden food are readily available as an almost immediate "anxiety fix." Weight gain, particularly in the first years of college, is common with not only periods of restriction, but also excessive exercise often used as the remedy. Thus, during these important years, binge eating disorder and exercise bulimia may emerge with greater frequency.

You are probably already aware that the progression of an eating disorder doesn't always follow the same pattern. For most patients, the disorder begins with simple disordered eating and, toward the end of high school and during college, rapidly escalates. Some patients can be defined as anorexic, bulimic, binge eaters, or exercise bulimics, but I firmly believe this is far too simplistic. If, like Lisa, you have experienced a mix of anorexia, bulimia, binge eating, or exercise bulimia at different points in your life, different seasons (perhaps bulimia in winter and anorexia in summer) or in different settings (i.e., different forms in the school setting than on vacations home), this is not unusual. As the years progress, without treatment, alternation in form may surely occur as the struggle for control intensifies. What is clear is that there is really no set norm with one category of eating disorder being safer, healthier, or more "effective" than any other. All are dangerous and life threatening. It's, of course, not as common, but an eating disorder can also begin in young adulthood or adulthood or even in later life, often at periods of high stress or acute transition. We're never safe!

Self-regulation

Self-regulation bears brief mentioning. In high school, life tends to follow a regular and predictable pattern. There is a time to get up, go to school, and come home. There is a time to eat, sleep, and spend on outside activities and with friends. Frequently, there is a set time for meals, and mom or someone at home prepares meals. Laundry is done, the house is maintained, and often transportation is provided. There is little need to self-regulate or even to learn how. Life is essentially mapped out. The years following high school present a totally different picture. All areas of life need redefining and regulating. For many of my eating-disordered patients, self-regulation is not well developed. With control and certainty being important areas, self-regulation becomes an anxiety-provoking task. In addition, lack of sleep due to increased life demands leads to fatigue and makes self-regulation even more difficult. The fatigue itself may lead to binge eating. Self-regulation of food becomes a primary and often difficult task.

The F Word—Food

The college years are often the first time in a student's life that they are required to choose when, where, and what they are going to eat. This can be quite overwhelming. In high school, others usually monitored food. Binge eating was frequently carefully planned so that the required food was available. In college, disordered or binge eating becomes easy. You are surrounded by food constantly. Roommates are constantly eating, and pizzas are ordered for late-night energy. Pretzels, cookies, and candy bars are a quick reward for long, hard study hours. Some sorority houses may employ their own fancy cooks;

there is a dining hall with an abundance of food, vending machines, and often a food court. There is an abundance of fried food, high-carbohydrate food, and unlimited desserts. Previously forbidden foods are continuously within arms reach. For some, a new sign of independence is just to let go and eat. For others, like Lisa, attempts at self-regulation lead to panic, with binge eating followed by restriction and/or excessive exercise, and so the cycle continues.

In addition, as we see with Lisa, students are under tremendous pressure to achieve both academically and socially. Students are often faced with managing life responsibilities and problems for the first time, and for which they are ill prepared. The stress is enormous. Life feels out of control. High-calorie, high-carbohydrate food is a cheap, fast, and simple comfort strategy that really does, at least temporarily, work. Food quickly becomes the stress-management technique of choice.

ILLUSIONS OF THINNESS AND OTHER FAIRY TALES

Culture, society, and stage of life transitions are essential stones and bricks in the building of an eating disorder. But one essential element is missing—the mortar that holds the stones and bricks together. In the development of an eating disorder, this mortar centers on the complex set of rapidly emerging cognitive and perceptual distortions that I discussed earlier. These distortions solidify an elaborate and growing system that not only keeps the eating disorder, but to a significant degree life itself, in a fragile balance with the illusion that everything is in order and in place. What is even more complex is that initially this elaborate system appears to have enormous and very real payoffs. As the eating disorder progresses, these fairy tales and all of the beliefs and actions surrounding them take greater and greater hold. These distortions initially seem to the person with an eating disorder completely real, true, and like the fairy tales of childhood providing unending happiness, the payoffs of being thin. If you are in the early stages of an eating disorder you, too, may still believe in these fairy tales and they may indeed seem very real and true. If you are in the later stages of an eating disorder, you have likely watched as this unstable mortar crumbled. You have realized that this fairy tale will not have a happy ending.

Fairy Tale 1: If I'm Thin, Everything Will Be Perfect

What is this great dream that we are taught from the earliest age? What is this illusion that leads so many people to place thinness above almost all else in their lives, including their health? What are the payoffs of thinness? The answers are both simple and complex. Early in her diary, Lisa wants to "look and feel terrific." Although our common sense tells us that this may be a rather vague and illusive dream, and we're not quite sure just what "terrific" means, nonetheless we fully and completely understand Lisa's feelings. Quite simply, people, especially females, from the earliest age are led to believe that, if they are thin enough, everything and anything is possible, and my patients, like Lisa, believe this with an almost unimaginable and tenacious intensity. If they can only be thin enough, they WILL look and feel terrific. If they are thin, they will have it "all" and that "all," even if they can't clearly define it, will be great. Even after Lisa is euphoric at reaching 115 pounds (less than a ten-pound loss from her usual weight), she writes:

"I want to have no stomach.
I want a little butt.
I want skinny fingers.
I want a thin face.
I want firm boobs.
I want a small waist.
In other words—*I want it all.*
GO FOR IT!!!"

Thus, the payoff of being thin is having it all. Thinness will bring success, happiness, popularity, boyfriends, and a great life. No matter how wildly the world around you is spinning out of control, if you are thin enough, you will be in control. If you are thin enough, you will be sought after and admired. Food restriction means strength, and, as we've seen, Lisa is restricting more than ever to maintain the weight loss, by drinking only cans of liquid protein. Thin means perfect. Thin means secure. Thin means powerful. Thin means sexual. THIN MEANS BEING LOVED.

There's reason for the euphoria Lisa has already experienced a few days prior to that writing. Why, a week out of high school and months before even starting college, she's already gotten her dream job at a television station, beating out 3,000 others—a fact she lets us know has at least something to do with the size-three pants she was wearing during the interview and the newfound confidence she has from the less-than-ten-pound weight loss, which she is also confusing with self-discovery. Just a few weeks after that, payoff number two walks onto one of the television sets in the form of a six-foot-two, blond, blue-eyed actor/model who immediately asks Lisa out and begins to sweep her off her feet. What else could this be but a true payoff from weight loss? Unfortunately, it is true, the world does often pay off for that. That gorgeous guy didn't know Lisa yet when he asked her out. He asked out the girl who had compelled herself to fit into a preconceived mold, and in that case it worked. That's why this is such a trap: There are payoffs, and they become addictive.

Therefore, it's not surprising in light of both the perceived and often very real payoffs that no price is thought to be too great in your quest for the perfect body. What is even more complex is that when the weight is lost, initially you may look better. That is real. Like Lisa, in the beginning, you may find yourself more outgoing and self-confident with many new successes. Friends may be more attracted to you and the dreamed-about boyfriend may appear as a result of the weight loss. With these initial, and what needs to be stressed is the word *initial*, powerful reinforcements the illusions become more entrenched. For Lisa, her new job success and handsome boyfriends were attributed entirely to her new body, and the quest for thinness intensified. More thinness meant more payoffs and intensified her feelings that thinness is everything.

Fairy Tale 2: If I'm Thin, I Will Be Happy

If thinness is everything, then happiness is a big piece of that pie. Those with eating disorders often become euphoric with weight loss. Lisa's stream of euphoric writing is a magnifying glass into this type of thinking:

"My life is consistently wonderful. That is not to say that everything is coming up roses. I am the rose. It may be raining upon me. The ground around me may turn to mud. I may be left to grow alone, yet, I, myself, remain calm, peaceful, strong, stable, and subtly beautiful. I am full of pride. I have done a great thing by losing weight, and continuing to do so," is just one of her many elated statements related to her weight loss.

Many of my patients describe a state of euphoria as they reach lower and lower weights. They describe all of the feelings that Lisa exudes. Focus is on the good things that are happening and the intense sense of control they are feeling. All negative feelings and thoughts are shelved. If you have an eating disorder, you are only too aware of this happy stage. The fairy tale of happily ever after is a powerful illusion that sets a powerful trap. Unfortunately, the happiness quickly disappears.

Fairy Tale 3: If I'm Thin, I Will Be Popular

For many caught in these cycles, one of the biggest draws of thinness is popularity. This fairy tale is a complex one. Moving away to college for most people means all new friends. Friends are important. Starting over is not always easy. Everyone worries about being accepted and fitting in. Many girls believe that the only way they will be accepted is if they are thin. Unfortunately, society tends to reinforce this belief. There is a big payoff to being thin. In the post-high school period, thinness will tend for some to bring increased admiration and greater ease in establishing new friendships. Therefore, it is not unusual for girls to find the summer before college a dieting extravaganza, in which they lose vast amounts of weight. Unfortunately, due to many factors, maintaining this weight loss the first year of college can be difficult, if not impossible. Since thin means popular and friendships are key, the cycle begins.

In addition, the new college student may no longer live in a family, but now live surrounded by other girls. Many of these girls, like many of their high school friends, will also be preoccupied with diet and weight. It is "in" to be on a diet, and diets, weight, and exercise make conversation easy. For many of my eating-disordered patients, comparing themselves to the other girls around them in terms of body size and weight is a daily preoccupation. They are acutely aware of the weight of their roommates, classmates, and dorm mates or sorority sisters, and compare their weight to others. Their friendship choices may be based on weight, just as they perceive others as choosing them because of their body size. In reality, entrance into a popular club or sorority may in part depend on appearance and body shape. As Lisa loses more and more weight, she writes: "I have never been this popular. I could never even imagine being this popular."

Lisa is being noticed and sought after and attributes all of this to her weight loss and new body shape. Her dieting behavior is thus reinforced, and the trap tightens. What Lisa is only beginning to realize is that she is not as happy as she thinks, and feels some confusion and sense of loss. For now, she has friends, but as the eating disorder progresses, the self-imposed demands and rituals, as well as the increasing secrecy, shame, and guilt will cause Lisa to isolate. Before long (in fact, well before this now-triumphant freshman college year ends), she will find herself strangely alone. The ending to this fairy tale is not popularity but shame, guilt, self-imposed isolation, and aloneness.

Fairy Tale 4: If I'm Thin, I Will Be Loved

When Lisa noted she was more popular than she ever dreamed, she primarily meant with members of the opposite sex. This is typical of the fairy tales surrounding becoming thin. Some boyfriends are more attracted! And, then for most with eating disorders, all of the conflicting feelings about sex and sexuality begin to emerge. We will quickly see this with Lisa, especially as she begins to realize that anxiety about sexuality may be much more of a stress than was her distorted feelings about her body. With my anorectic patients, what may emerge is numbness, fear, withdrawal, and disassociation; with bulimics, I often see more multiple relationships, some wild sexual acting out, and then shame, guilt, and withdrawal, and increased binging and purging as the relationship intensifies. Many have significant issues with showing their nude body. In addition for some, as for Lisa, this awakens unresolved dependency issues, as they lose themselves in relationships and try to be all that the partner wants them to be. This increases the fear of dissolution of the relationship and brings up issues of the dissolution of the self. As you may already know, it is a very different way to live.

Fairy Tale 5: I Am In Control

As Lisa's measurements and numbers on the scale move steadily downward, she writes:

"Life is mine. Life is challenging. Life is adventure. Life is acceptance. Life is calm, serene, and peaceful. . . . Life is courage, strength, and confidence. Life is joy beyond ecstasy. Life is love, simple in its complex intricacies. I have taken the reins of my life in my own hands. I grabbed control."

Although these words may at first glance seem overdramatic, most with eating disorders feel exactly the same way. As you watch the numbers on the scale go steadily downward, you probably feel ecstatic and even grandiose, believing firmly that you are not only in control of your body, but also the world around you.

In all eating disorders, complete control over thoughts, feelings, actions, and, most of all, control over the body is an essential part of the mortar. The illusion is, "if I am in control of my body, I am in control of my world." I am in control and I can maintain control no matter what the circumstances. The fairy tale is, "if I can only continue to maintain control, all else wonderful will follow forever." The reality is that this is an impossible dream exacting an enormous price.

Let's look for a minute at just how this control is maintained. Judy Asner, a fellow eating-disorders specialist, recently eloquently and simply described this to me about her patients. This is what I am seeing every day. Those who have eating disorders completely organize their lives around food. Food, as the organizing principal of life, determines their thoughts, feelings, and, equally importantly, their actions. It determines where they go, what they do, and how they spend much of their time. For most, the night before or early morning hours are spent in planning the day in detail, figuring out set times for daily body measuring, weigh-ins, exercise, and the intricate details of how, when, where, and how much food will be consumed. Frequently, exercise is factored into the picture. This becomes an exhausting and time-consuming daily task. As the eating disorder progresses, all other life activities and friendships become secondary, a part of the picture only as time permits. Life as they knew it in the past begins to change and narrow. This is key!

Lisa expressed this kind of obsessive planning earlier in her diary. She was already laying in bed trying to go to sleep, when she instead—as she told me she often did—got up to exercise and wrote, "While I was in bed I was thinking, I can't wait until tomorrow to get back on track after blowing it today by overeating. Then I thought I could still get something done tonight. I'm glad I did. . . . Well, I just danced around like crazy and I feel great. . . . Before, I felt lazy and fat like I wouldn't be able to get back into it. Well, I did great. I want to do my workout again before bed. Tomorrow, here I come!"

In her diary, we see Lisa maintaining an ongoing pep talk with herself each time her control weakens. "I am strong, I am special, I can do it. Life is beautiful. I AM IN CONTROL." This pep talk is essential in the maintenance of an eating disorder. In the ongoing internal dialogue, all negative thoughts and feelings like sadness, fear, confusion, and pain are replaced by positive messages. Each time control weakens, the positive dialogue becomes stronger and more positive. This was clear every time Lisa wrote:

"You are strong.
You will make it.
You can roll with the punches
You are a winner."

"I will be what I will to be
I will do what I will to do
I want to be!
I am.
I love life."

The messages also become more pervasive, and soon the ongoing dialogue that was set up to maintain control becomes more and more frequent and out of control. For some, the head messages are so intense they may feel as if they are going crazy, even though that is not the case. As we can note in the second vignette, there may be a vast discrepancy between Lisa's head messages and her current reality. Grandiosity and magical thinking, which I talked about in Chapter 3, help to maintain this as well as many of the other illusions.

Although consciously those with eating disorders describe a feeling of mastery and control over much of the world around them when they are controlling their food intake and exercise, they are also acutely aware of another set of feelings. That is the intense fear that if they loosen these controls even slightly, they will begin rapidly gaining weight. This can be an all-consuming and terrifying fear. What they may be less aware of is the much more significant, vague, underlying fear that if they loosen controls at all, something very bad will happen. At that point, they have not yet realized that their very life has become organized around the eating disorder, and they believe if the eating disorder is taken away they will have nothing, be nothing, and evaporate.

Fairy Tale 6: Thin Is Good, Thinner Is Better

This mindset couldn't be clearer than when Lisa, who has now, through virtual starvation and forced exercise, dropped to 112 pounds, decides she wants to lose more and defines this journey to her desired 103 pounds (or lower if she gives it "serious consideration") as "self-discovery":

"Another crossroads along the path to self-discovery: I find that I can't just settle for being 'thin' or 'trim' or 'fit' or 'in good shape.' What is it, then, that I want, and is it realistic? . . . I want to be a knockout! I want to be in great shape! I want to have a terrific figure. . . . I feel my potential is immense. Why stop at an A- when you have A+ potential."

This is, of course, the rub. If you or a loved one are like Lisa, or the millions who have eating disorders, thin is never thin enough. You will be chasing a gold ring that is constantly just out of reach. This throws you into a no-win and thoroughly exhausting psychological state and often a physical state that may involve seesawing between weight loss (as you follow your forced plan) and weight gain (as you inevitably fall off the wagon, as we have seen Lisa do). So Lisa, always the perfectionist, reasons, if thin is good, thinner is better. This is a pattern I see in most of my patients. As the numbers on the scale decrease, thinking becomes more and more distorted and weight goals get lower and lower, until there is no ability to distinguish reality. Thin is never thin enough.

As far as we know, Lisa's weight never reached a critically dangerous stage. Other patients of mine have not been as lucky. A patient writes: "Being thin seems to never be enough. When you're anorexic and are very thin your mind will play tricks on you. You'll keep looking in the mirror and never be satisfied. I can remember in college when I was at my almost lowest weight, 78 pounds, and honestly did not believe that I was thin. I wasn't at all scared of the fact that I was on the brink of death. I was more scared that my hair was falling out. I had severe chest pains all the time. I couldn't sleep at all. I had to wake up an hour earlier to dress myself and get ready for class since I had no energy. I walked so slowly I couldn't get up the steps. It wasn't until then that I realized that other people were staring at me. When I could no longer exercise as hard and as long as I wanted to, I really became upset. Before I could run unending seven minute miles and now it hurt to walk."

"Anorexia is so crazy. You begin with a number that you want to weigh and somewhere, somehow, along the line the number keeps changing. Every time you achieve it the number gets lower and lower to the point you are hospitalized or die. I look back now and can't believe I almost died."

What is even more frightening is that many outsiders tend to continue to reinforce the weight loss. "You're still losing weight. How do you do it? You look great." As I noted in my last chapter, Lisa told me that even the hospital-based registered dietitian, who should have been trained to pick up the signs of eating disorders, gave 112-pound Lisa just such a stunned compliment. Lisa had returned to figure out how to control her low weight, which seemed to be spiraling out of control whenever she ate a morsel.

Even at very low and clearly unhealthy body weights, friends and family will rarely confront you, and even if they did, you would probably block them out and not hear what they were saying. You would not let their opinions take hold of your own beliefs. You will see Lisa struggling with this pattern for the next months, until she seeks help that, as far as she is concerned, is for her eating problem, until she begins to note the problem, amazingly, has little to do with eating and everything to do with self-concept.

THINNESS—UGLY REALITY

Fairy tales are created out of so many things—culture, the environment, expectations, and even our dreams. Fairy tales are created out of friendships and the basic need to be loved. For so many of my patients there was also a lack of intimacy and identity at crucial developmental stages. All of these parts had a crucial role in the formation of their eating disorders. Getting back to my analogy of a house being built: in childhood the foundation of the house is poured. In adolescence some 2x4s are added. By early adulthood the walls have gone up. What is necessary to hold this house together is a framework and mortar. If there is no framework, the house will fall. Thus, in all of the above areas, but in particular in the areas of intimacy and identity, the need to create a framework. The existing framework is a huge dysfunctional system centered around the body and thinness that gives them a sense of integration and boundaries and helps them make sense of the world. It tells them what they need to do to be loved, successful, and in control. It is supported by an elaborate system of beliefs, including the myths and fairy tales I have been describing.

If you have an eating disorder, like Lisa, you may begin to break down, be unable to function, and be terribly confused and upset when you quickly realize that your hard-won goal of thinness doesn't shine as bright as those first heady days, weeks, or months. If you had been obsessed with thinness and how it would make you feel, your mind will find it hard to accept conflicting feelings.

"Why pull yourself down like today?" Lisa writes after binging before slipping her now-perfect body into a bikini at a party surrounded by television's beautiful people. "Why couldn't you have just gone to Pierre's going away party? You swam. You sat by the pool in your skimpy bathing suit, and you knew you looked good. Yes, it was a lot different from parties from years before. Yes, you felt like a different person. Yes, it was weird. . . . Why did you have to stop at that supermarket on the way? No, two candy bars might not have seemed like a big binge before, but now it's huge. And on the way home? A pint of ice cream is right back down your old path. Things were supposed to be different now. At 112 pounds, things are supposed to be different."

The thing is, and it's important, things are not different because those with eating disorders who change only their weight, or simply try valiantly to control their eating, are overlooking the real problems. Help is needed to break free of this pattern. Many people with eating disorders are high-achieving perfectionists. (Of course, not all are.) Unfortunately, as you will see Lisa do in the next diary chapters, most high-achieving perfectionists with eating disorders, without realizing there are urgent underlying problems, think they can solve the problem themselves and go to huge extremes to do so. Later, though, you will witness firsthand as Lisa finally gets professional help, and I'll make suggestions along the way so that you, too, can best find help for yourself or a loved one.

It may be a relief, for the first time, to understand why you (or a loved one) are behaving in a certain way. If you or a loved one has an eating disorder, you may already have been aware of the myths we have described. In fact, you may still believe that some of them are real. You have probably also created other myths and fairy tales and believe them to be equally true. Even though you may not believe it now, ever so slowly and imperceptibly, the mortar will begin to crumble for you as it did for Lisa.

As you struggle to regain control, you will find yourself more and more out of control and may even wonder just what it is you are really controlling. Then, like Lisa, your November 1 will arrive: "Mom. Oh, mom, please help me. That's what I said today. Finally I had to tell someone I needed help. I can't take it anymore . . . there is something wrong with me." Our main motivation in this book is so that you, like Lisa, might not only recognize the problem, but also seek needed help. What I'll talk about in my upcoming chapter is why the first help you might employ—your own—has severe built-in limitations, and why it's crucial to search out qualified professional assistance. You'll see some of those very real-life limitations in Lisa's next diary chapters, as she "white-knuckles it" before descending into "momentary hell."

5. Limbo

18 TO 19 YEARS OLD

What's in store for me? Can I control it? Why did I leave school mid-term? The reasons, I have a feeling, are more complex than I seem to be experiencing. Do I still love myself? Where's that feeling of ecstasy that I had in the summer when I first lost the weight? I want it back. I've got to try. I may not have answers, but I can't give up. No matter what, I'm going to do it. Confidence. That's what I need. I can and will help myself. Ecstasy, here I come.

This is the most important thing in my life.
Weight: 120 pounds

FOOD:

Breakfast:		**Dinner:**	
1 slice diet bread	50	3 oz. bologna	210
1 tbsp. peanut butter	90	12 wheat thins	70
1 cup non-fat milk	80		
½ grapefruit	40	**Total Calories**	856
Lunch:			
1 bagel	140		
2 oz. chicken	120		
1 apple	40		
diet dressing	16		

EXERCISE

hula hoops: 400 times	workout: at home
jump ropes: 200 times	swim at club: 40 laps
jump rope workouts: 2	bed exercises
television exercise show	bike: 2.5 miles
workout: at club	

NOVEMBER 16

MEASUREMENTS
(My "New Life" Program Begins)

Waist: 24"   Hips: $34\frac{1}{2}$"
Bust: 35"   Abdomen: $31\frac{1}{2}$"
Thighs: $20\frac{1}{2}$"   Lower leg: $12\frac{1}{2}$"
Upper arm: 10"   Calf: 7"

NOVEMBER 17

"New Life" Day One
Weight: $115\frac{1}{2}$ pounds

FOOD

Breakfast: **Dinner:**
1 wheat bread   3 oz. chicken
1 tbsp. peanut butter $\frac{1}{2}$ baked potato
1 cup non-fat milk   mixed veggies
$\frac{1}{2}$ grapefruit   1 tbsp. soy sauce
                                                 1 tbsp. oil
Lunch: 1 glass iced tea
1 wheat bread
2 oz. turkey
1 glass iced tea

EXERCISE

bed exercises   pool exercises
morning routine   evening routine
face-ups   face-ups
hula hoop, 250 times   weights
bike: 1 mile   jump ropes: 100
workout   jump rope workout
swim: 40 laps

NOVEMBER 17

Sooo, this is life. Very interesting, confusing stuff. I like myself. A lot. I want to say that first, because I can see that's what it takes. Everything else will follow. I can and will make it. Things won't always be easy, but I think I am learning to cope.

School. I'm really sick of talking about it. What has been done has been done. No regrets. Life and living lie ahead. I'll be working my television studio page job for the next few months and then start broadcasting and journalism classes at Cal State, Northridge. So, I'll get my degree from there. I can't go back to USC after losing all that money and all my scholarships. Well, Perry couldn't believe that I, the straight-A student, should drop out my first semester of college. But then, he doesn't know the real reason. I love him, and it's always getting better. I will soon be seeing the psychiatrist recommended through Mom's doctor. I think he has a specialty in eating disorders.

Something happened tonight. I'm upset, so everything I say may be regarded as ludicrous and an overreaction later. It's about my father. I don't know if I'm all that wild about him as a person. I love him; he's smart. But I don't like his perspective, where "he's coming from." He called me selfish and irresponsible. It was something to do with the car. He said, "You know, maybe I'll decide Mom needs the car and you won't be able to use it anymore to drive into Hollywood every day for work." If only he knew how miserable I am. In one breath he said I could pay him half my savings account and buy the car. In the next he asked why in the world I would give up a deal where I could use a car for free except for gas. If only he knew how miserable I am.

I know what's really important. Keeping my peace of mind. Without it nothing works. I need it in order to live one day at a time.

That's not selfishness. That's survival.

NOVEMBER 19

Forget this, I am buying the car.

He's, of course, going to say there's no way he said he'd sell it to me for half my bank account. Who'd sell a $15,000 car for $2,500, he'll ask?

Who'd be stupid enough not to buy a cute little $15,000 car for $2,500 is what I've been asking myself? Why just drive, in fear of losing your right to drive, when you can own? I'd rather pay repairs and insurance and know that no one can take it away from me.

LATER: Well, first he said exactly what I said he would, "I never said that. That would be ridiculous." Then he said he'd think about it. Later he said, "Yes, if you want to give me half the money in your bank account, I'll sell you the car."

NOVEMBER 20

I commit, I commit, I commit.

Others can do it.

I can do it. As one writer put it, I have given up the right to overeat. Binge, that is. I love myself too much. I have faith in me. I am capable of it.

Eating a dessert or treat is not compulsive overeating.

I commit.

Perry,

I love you. No point in beating around the bush. Love is not a commitment, but a feeling. The two do not have to go hand in hand.

So don't get scared. I don't want anything from you. I know I seem like an incredibly easy person to please. Maybe I am. It's not that I don't want anything from you, it's just that I'm satisfied with what you feel comfortable in giving.

Giving is not only *things*. That's unimportant, and, in the long run, doesn't matter much. People who can give of themselves and share their hopes, dreams, problems, and everyday trivialities are the biggest givers.

So, I think you're a wonderful person. I think we're both wonderful. Two people who could have anyone they wanted and pick each other. I think that's the healthiest kind of relationship.

I felt like saying it for a long time, but I was afraid. I still am, a little. Over the past months, I've seen us both changing and growing. I like the results, but I know we've still got a way to go before we're through.

On what you said about making decisions: I make them. Sometimes they're not verbal, but I would never just go along with something sexual or otherwise. What I do, I do because I want to. I decided a long time ago, when you love someone, what you do is right.

I just don't want you to feel badly. Sometimes it's hard for me to express myself. Just know that it's more my nature to be passive than aggressive.

Until now, I've been playing it safe. There comes a point, though, when you've already given up enough that playing it safe doesn't seem as necessary. I feel relieved.

So now you know how I feel. You probably already did. It calls for no reaction, response, or answer.

I'm happy with the way things are right now. I'm happy with you.

(*Never Sent*)

I am a yo-yo. I don't want to be. My life is either terribly up or terribly down. Where is the balance? Where am I? Uncertainty looms. I don't want to be a yo-yo anymore.

I am grabbing control again.

Live.

LATER: All of a sudden I am very scared. I am a prisoner. I think about it all the time. How I act, how I think, what I do. It is in my every thought. It looms twenty-four hours a day. Every day. Whether I am eating sensibly or overeating, it is always there.

Who am I kidding? I'm not free. I'm locked up. It's always there, either in the front or back of my mind. Controlling me.

What do I do?

DECEMBER 4

Starting bloated weight: $120\frac{1}{2}$

DECEMBER 5

All liquid to clean out system and drop water weight.

Dec. 4	Dec. 5	Dec. 6	Dec. 7	Dec. 8	Dec. 9	Dec. 10
$120\frac{1}{2}$	$119\frac{1}{2}$	$117\frac{1}{2}$				I blew it!
Dec. 11	Dec. 12	Dec. 13	Dec. 14	Dec. 15	Dec. 16	Dec. 17

What It Takes
Balanced low-cal food plan
Exercise
Positive thinking

Ideal Exercise Plan
morning routine
bed exercises
face-ups (2)
100 jump ropes
jump rope workout
200 hula hoops
weights
bike: 1 mile
workout
swim: 30 laps
pool exercises
evening routine

Positive Thinking Plan
Feel good about you.
Think "up" thoughts.
Make the most of situations.
Like you.

One day at a time.
Let yourself relax.
Let yourself feel.

DECEMBER 6

I am all alone.

I am not going back to that guy. I put a message on his service that I was canceling my next appointment and would not be back. Three times: $475 of my mom's dollars—no dad involved—and he asks me about my infant days. Fine, but every time I'd leave, I'd stop at McDonald's and Jack in the Box and Arby's. By the time I'd get home, I'd be bloated and numb.

This last time did it. He said, you know, Lisa, I notice the few times you've come, you've worn button blouses that buckle a little. He's there looking at my buckling button and asks me if there's anything regarding the size of my breasts and men I'd like to tell him. He hopes he's not embarrassing me, but the thought just occurred to him.

What does this 50-year-old, plush-officed person know about me and my problems?

As always, I am all alone.

DECEMBER 9

And so it comes to an end, the year, and another era of self. I guess I should also say a beginning. Honestly, however, I must say that things are not clear.

What does seem clear at this point is that I would like to weigh between 110 and 115 pounds instead of 120 pounds because that is where I look and feel best.

Last summer, after high school graduation, I lost weight by getting ill and then drinking liquid protein. The weight came off quickly, but when I began eating, what happened? I have to learn to deal with this realistically. Everything is relative.

I need compassion.

I am at a good place.

I love myself. Period. The way I am.

I choose to change.

DECEMBER 21

I want to write it down, so I don't forget. Although I'm sure the best is still yet to come, *wow*, attention from the opposite sex is at a peak. Maybe it's just that for once the attention is coming from very desirable people. Three. All nice-looking. In different ways, and to varying degrees, handsome, actually. All three are extremely intelligent, again in different ways, and all are extremely interesting/fascinating.

I know I love Perry. I think I'm in love with him. But this experimentation is wonderful.

My first television "wrap" party was great! At least I felt great, dancing with stars—TV, music, film stars. And Brent, my until-now-flirting page friend, is full of passion for me, thinks I'm gorgeous, and loves to have me on his arm. Now we've crossed a little over that platonic line. Just take everything slowly.

Thought I was going to tell Greg to get lost and look what happened. Everything's better than ever. I still left the party with him. I think he's sweet and would like to believe everything he said when we finally spoke honestly.

Whatever! These sweeties have one thing in common, good taste.

DECEMBER 25

Turning point. My life is about to begin. I am beginning. Last year about this time, I felt as if my life journey was beginning. It was. So what's starting now? The path toward self-honesty. That's different. God, is it going to take work. Day by day. Minute by minute. I can do it. I believe in myself. I really do. I don't have the answers. I never will. But that's part of the excitement; I don't need answers.

All I need is the desire to seek.

DECEMBER 26

This is a matter of life and death, or more appropriately between living and non-living. Maybe it's not a physical, literal death, but certainly it's an emotional death. I'm binging and purging myself to death.

I opt for life. Every day that option must be renewed. It is not automatic. I've got it. Right now I'm uncovering and discovering it.

LATER: I'm writing this so that next week when I'm feeling good I will not forget how I feel now.

I *feel* fat. I feel ugly. My skin is breaking out. I feel like I look just awful. This is going to end.

It is. I will.

DECEMBER 27

I am not going
to forget this
nightmare of a
life.

DECEMBER 30

So, I learned something. As if I didn't know. The strange thing is that I really didn't. One bite *is* all it takes. God, I really only intended to take one, to prove to myself that I could. I guess if you just don't have that first bite, ever. I'm not just dealing with tomorrow or next week, I'm dealing with my life.

I'm not going to punish myself by not eating, that's just part of the same vicious cycle. In fact, I can use this as a learning experience.

I have a right to my life.

JANUARY 3

Resolution: to live happily and healthily *and* to be consciously aware of it.

I looked in the mirror. I talked to myself. I watched myself. I saw what others seem to see, a very pretty girl. Why is it that I usually carry a different image in my mind?

I liked what I saw even though it wasn't what I particularly wanted to see. Today wasn't easy, but I took it as it came, and I made it.

JANUARY 7

Today is January 7 and I feel wonderful. There is a subtly beautiful feeling tingling just beneath my skin.

The difference, true, is only a few pounds, but it could be hundreds. What causes this shift in moods? A sense of non-being turns to a sense of well-being.

JANUARY 8

Well, thank God I could get back in. Any student can take up to a one-year leave without losing student status. I just registered like nothing happened.

I kept saying to myself these last few months, "Hey, there was a reason you picked this school regarding your career and future. You put some thought into this decision. Are you just going to throw it all away?"

I'd be standing on the audience lines at work as a television studio page talking to tourists and they'd ask me where I went to school, and I realized I wanted to say USC. Not any other school, just USC. I finally thought, there's no way I'm going to let this thing eat away my chance at the education of my choice.

So, I'm back. I found an apartment off campus with a girl from Singapore. I like my part of the apartment. It's big. It looks like things might work out after all.

JANUARY 13

I'm lying in my bed in my room. In my half of the apartment.

So far, so good.

I'm taking things, life, one day at a time.

I can really say that at this moment, right now, I feel happy, pleased.

Way to go.

JANUARY 18

WEIGHT RECORD (Weekly)

Date:	1/11	1/18	1/25	2/1	2/8
Weight:	120.5	118.5			
Weekly Loss: 2.0				Total Loss: 2.0	

JANUARY 18

Hips: 35"   Bust: 35½"
Waist: 24½"   Thighs: 21"

JANUARY 21

Today is a landmark in my life. Another journey is beginning. I am ready. I am dedicating my life to me by abstinence from compulsive overeating. I have made a commitment to myself. I like myself enough. I am going to take life a minute at a time. It takes what it takes. I am committed to following a balanced eating and exercise program. My life *depends* upon acceptance and execution of these commitments.

I have just closed and locked the door behind me. Ah, the fresh air. The fog makes it impossible to see what lies ahead. It is my life.

JANUARY 22

Today, I turned 19 and I'm ready to embark. To participate. To live.

Yesterday, I made a commitment. But who am I today? In some ways I don't know. I am pretty. I do have good friends (a list to look back on someday and wonder about): Perry, Noreen, Cheri, Bob, Greg.

I like myself. I wear a size seven.

6. White-Knuckling It

19 YEARS OLD

I have reached the point of no return. Abstinence from compulsive overeating is the most important thing in my life, without exception.

My old life is just that, my old life. I will not forget the desperation. However, that is not now, and all that matters is now. Now. It is the present I have given to myself, present moment living.

I realized that my life is my choice. Whether I was consciously aware of it or not, I was choosing to feel miserable.

I do not choose that any longer. I do not need to continue it.

I felt like a snake almost ready to shed an outer skin, a skin that served no purpose and yet was hanging on, still remaining part of my life.

The skin has been shed. The nightmare is over. I can make my life over.

It *is* over, because I choose it to be. I have that power. It has no power. I have always had the power. Now I realize that, and I choose to utilize and channel it positively.

Life at last!

"Point of No Return" Day 1

Breakfast:		Dinner:	
1 wheat bread	70	3 oz. Chicken	180
1 tbsp. peanut butter	90	$\frac{1}{2}$ cup brown rice	70
1 cup non-fat milk	90	veggies	30
	250	12 grapes	40
Lunch:		1 tbsp. soy sauce	30
1 apple	45		350
1 apple	45	**Total:**	690 calories
	90		

"Point of No Return" Day 6
Weight: 119 pounds

Breakfast:			**Dinner:**	
1 slice wheat bread	70		1 oz. turkey ham	65
1 tbsp. peanut butter	90		2 oz. cheese	140
1 cup non-fat milk	90		diet dressing	25
$\frac{1}{2}$ grapefruit	40		1 slice wheat bread	70
	290		cooking oil	20
				320

Lunch:				
1 turkey hot dog	100		**Total:**	905 calories
1 oz. cheese	60			
$\frac{1}{2}$ small potato	70			
1 tbsp. diet dressing	25			
12 grapes	40			
	295			

LATER: This is hard, leaving an old way of life for a new one. Remnants of the old keep pulling and beckoning; they are so ingrained. However, all that's left is that ingrained feeling. The reasons for the eating behavior are no longer here, as they were for the past six years! Yes! At least six, maybe even as many as eleven, blocked out.

Minute by minute, I am creating a new life for myself. I'm worth it.

"Point of No Return" Day 10
English Class Journal
3:30–3:45 P.M.

I had an experience yesterday. Usually, I would put an adjective before "experience," however, I am confused as to just what that adjective should be. I know that what happened affected me, but I'm not sure whether or not it should have.

A woman's voice on the phone at work asked, "May I leave a message for Greg Butler?" Yes. Of course. I wanted to find out who it was, his mother?

"Just tell him Jenny called. I'll call him later." Who calls to leave a message like that?

"OK. Anything else?" That's what I wanted to hear, more. I don't want to be left with "Jenny," that doesn't tell me anything.

"Yes, just tell him I love him."

What? I always wondered if there were others. Why shouldn't there have been? I'm on the verge of love with someone else. (And that's Perry, the same person I keep wondering if I love!) Why shouldn't some girl be in love with him? And yet, unrealistically, I always thought I was the only one.

I have no right to feel jealous or hurt or betrayed. And yet I do. It being my job to relay messages, I did. I wondered what to write.

I wrote it all. Better that he knows I know. Handing it to him, I couldn't look at him. My heart beat quick. He had to work late, in order, no doubt, to avoid our usual end of work "rap and kiss session."

I'm not sure what or how I feel. It was an experience. Period.

"Point of No Return" Day 11
English Class Journal
9:45–10:00 A.M.

Well, Perry just left again. This time, however, it was different. It wasn't a rushed, "My parents will wonder where I am, ha-ha." No parents. This time we pulled an "all-nighter."

Even though we've never "slept together," we've never slept together, literally, either. For me, it added a whole new dimension. How else would I have found out about those allergy-induced snores?

No matter how doubtful I am twenty-seven or twenty-eight days a month, these fifteen-hour rendezvous erase those doubts at least for fifteen hours. When near him, I feel love. I don't wonder. I don't question. I just experience, and feel like yelling it out, or whispering. I never do.

Those fifteen hours also confirm his love for me, at least in my mind. I can feel it seeping through his skin into mine. And yet he's been gone only minutes, and already I wonder.

I pretended we were on our honeymoon. I pretended this was our life together. Then I stopped pretending. I just floated.

English Class Journal
3:45–4:00 P.M.

I always thought there was a moment when life began, a starting point, turning eighteen, attending college, falling in love.

It wasn't until I turned eighteen, attended college, and fell in love that I realized the absurdity of my attitude. No outside event can cause a lasting, significant change. We can't depend on others or external events to make us happy. These can only enhance an already fulfilled individual. They do not create one.

I think it is true that happiness is "in your own back yard," mental back yard, that is. If you can't find it there, you won't find it anywhere. That's why happiness remains elusive to so many people, they search when all they have to do is breathe.

We are never powerless. We are never hopeless. We are always what we choose to be.

FEBRUARY 8

English Class Journal
6:15–6:30 P.M.

Love is confusing. At least, for me. Although I am still in the midst of my first encounter, I get the impression that this is an aspect of life marked by constant uncertainty, that never gets any easier.

One moment I feel quite sure that I am in love. The next moment I feel quite sure it is just infatuation, quasi-love or some other less intense emotion.

Then there are the times I'm absolutely sure Perry's in love with me. (Whenever we're together.) Most of the time, however, I am convinced that his motives are less than honorable. (Whenever we're apart.)

As soon as things gel and become clear in my mind, something, real or imagined, jolts my confidence back into a cloudy daze.

Oh well. I once read that only the insecure people seek security. I yearn for that security which will make me feel secure in my insecurity.

FEBRUARY 12

"Point of No Return" Day 14
Weight: 118 pounds

FEBRUARY 13

"Point of No Return" Day 15

FEBRUARY 14

"Point of No Return" Day 16
English Class Journal
9:00–9:15 A.M.

Valentine's Day. I'm sure many people get depressed on this day, the day for love, the day for being with your loved one. You can try and forget the significance of the fourteenth, perhaps, by not looking at the calendar. However, if you're alive and well, it's difficult to totally escape the reminders bombarding you through card stores, radio, television, newspapers, and just about every-where else.

Anyone lonely to begin with is doomed for an even greater onset of more of the same. Those with broken hearts must feel the pain more acutely.

FEBRUARY 14

English Class Journal
9:15–9:30 A.M.
"Without rain, there could be no rainbows."

Smile. Open your eyes wide to life. Experience. Breathe.
Give yourself rainbows. Let yourself go.

Close yourself up and you will wither.
Live one day at a time, minute by minute.
Create your own rainbows.

We are our own sunshine.
We can live on our own solar power.
A smile is a ray of sunlight.
Shine on.

FEBRUARY 15

"Point of No Return" Day 17
English Class Journal
2:35–2:50 P.M.
Last night. A landmark. A milestone. I denied an urge. *I didn't do it.* I didn't binge. Why? I'm not exactly sure, but I did want it to go down in recorded history.

I am kicking this thing once and for all. A destructive, emotional crutch, a crutch that's breaking apart. Because I'm breaking away.

I can walk.

For the first time, I can breathe. Never again to suffocate myself.

English Class Journal
2:55–3:10 P.M.
My Knight in shining armor,
My Prince Charming,
I used to dream of you.
Then I waited for you.
You were handsome.

You were brilliant.
Sweet,
Tender,
Jewish!
I couldn't understand where you were hiding.
I decided you were a figment of my imagination,
But, Perry, you were here all along.
I didn't recognize you at first.
You have helped me to fulfill my dreams.
I love you.

FEBRUARY 16

"Point of No Return" Day 18

FEBRUARY 17

"Point of No Return" Day 19

FEBRUARY 18

"Point of No Return" Day 20
I have found someone I can talk to. From an ad in the school newspaper I end up with the psychologist I dreamed I could meet. I saw her last month on the national TV talk show on which I work backstage. I wasn't working the day she was there; I saw her on the televised episode!

Well, I actually dreamed I could meet the patient who was with her.
Here was a woman on television talking about *my* problem. Even if I don't throw up, the similarities are too many, since I binge and then purge by starving or extreme calorie restriction, and forcing myself to exercise. I thought, if only I could talk to that patient, she would understand.

And here I make a call and I get the same psychologist. The ad said group therapy, but it looks like I might meet a while alone with her. What a difference from the other guy. Immediately, my first time there, I felt warmth and comfort and a *woman* I could relate to and respect.

FEBRUARY 19

"Point of No Return" Day 21
English Class Journal
8:00–8:15 A.M.
Restroom philosophy. This tiny cubicle is the only place of refuge on campus. The library was closed. I am alone. That is neither good nor bad. That is just a feeling of the moment.

These last few days have been the first time I've never had anyone to depend on, but myself. It's scary, yet invigorating. For the most part, I am on my own.

The turn of events with my car problems were anything but pleasant, and yet I managed. Am managing. I did not resort to that serpent crutch. Don't get me wrong. The urge to eat was there. Quite strong. I fought it. I'm not exactly sure how, but I fought it.

FEBRUARY 20

"Point of No Return" Day 22
English Class Journal
7:00–7:15 P.M.
"Many people
go from one thing
to another
searching for happiness,
but with each new venture
they find themselves
more confused and less happy
until they discover
that what they are
searching for
is inside themselves
and what will make them happy is sharing
their real selves with the ones
they love."
—*Anonymous*

I am lonely, I think. I don't feel terrific. I thought I would after not binging for so long. I'm tired. I'm not exactly sure what I want. I would like to wake up with a charge. Energy. Zest. Eager and ready to go. I would like to keep my mind clear, filled with positive thoughts. I would like to squeeze joy just by being me. Just from being alone. That would make the times with others more special.

I want to secrete a zest for living.

I have that capacity.

It's a matter of perspective and attitude.

Thought control. Present moment living.

FEBRUARY 21

"Point of No Return" Day 23
English Class Journal

10:05–10:20 A.M.

I don't like to complain. But, everybody needs an outlet, and all is not paradise in roommatesville. Listed below are some annoying traits:

Messy
- Her room (she's never unpacked)
- Her part of the kitchen
- Never puts away her dishes

Dog
- Supposed to be gone weeks ago
- I hate him
- Barks every morning when I get up
- Goes to bathroom on carpet
- I hate him

Makes me uncomfortable
- "Why you up so early"
- "Peanut butter make you fat"

Ignorance/Stupidity
- Not sure why, if it's a difference in our cultures, or if she's just dumb
- Desk lamp on kitchen table
- Dog on kitchen table
- Disgusting old food in refrigerator
- Trash
- Has only key, but never takes in mail

OK, so I got most of it out. Now, unless I am going to take specific action, I'm not going to waste my time on it.

FEBRUARY 21

English Class Journal
12:00–12:15 P.M.

Friends are important, providing perspectives, outlets, ears. Sometimes they are taken for granted.

A good friend is like a rare wine, long in the making, growing better and more priceless with time. It's better to sip and savor their company than gulp it down all at once.

Bob is my friend, someone I can talk with, someone who listens. He is a sincere, sweet, and sensitive person. Deep and intense. Our friendship was a fluke. A lucky fluke. The first person I met in college. One of the most important.

FEBRUARY 22

"Point of No Return" Day 24
DAILY FOOD PROGRAM

Breakfast:		Snack:	
1 nonfat milk	90	1 fruit	60
1 fruit	40		
1 bread	70	**Dinner:**	
1 meat	90	1 nonfat milk	90
		Vegetable	40
Lunch:		1 fruit	50
Vegetable	40	1 bread	70
1 fruit	55	3 meats	240
2 breads	140		
2 meats	160	**Total:**	1235 calories

No peanut butter.
Only one ounce of cheese per day.
Measure things when possible.
Do not eat beef.
Only one can of sugar-free soda per day.
Six glasses of water per day.
Do not leave anything out.

FEBRUARY 23 TO FEBRUARY 26

"Point of No Return" Day 25
"Point of No Return" Day 26
"Point of No Return" Day 27
"Point of No Return" Day 28

FEBRUARY 27

"Point of No Return" Day 29
I feel wonderful. Finally. Fitness. Energy. Vitality. This is great. The payoff from not binging.

I feel better than ever. It's worth it.

Here's to today and todays.

FEBRUARY 28

"Point of No Return" Day 30

I am in the process of learning to love my life, to love myself, unconditionally. I have been changing gradually. This has been the most remarkable thing I have done. In ways it's been powerful, in other ways subtle.

A month of abstinence from compulsive overeating.

I am learning to cope. My mind is clear.

I feel wonderfully terrific.

Spectacular.

LATER: English Class Journal
5:30–5:45 P.M.

I ate Chinese food today. Big deal? It was! Anything that has to do with controlled eating is a big deal for me. Controlled is the operative word. In the recent past I would have eaten the Chinese and everything else in sight (and out of it, too). Under the guise of having food that I enjoy, I would have set a trap, then the guilt would come, and a binge with it. So what's changed? I have. I still am. I took charge of the situation. Today, I thought it would be nice to have Chinese food. Not a single ulterior motive. I planned. I took precautions. Since I had a later breakfast I would skip lunch, just have a big apple when I got hungry, then I could have a combo lunch-dinner meal.

No guilt. Well, not really. Some of those old feelings are gnawing just under the surface. However, I know that they are just remnants of a past behavior to be ignored. It's getting easier. It's not easy. I've taken the liberty of writing my own fortune cookie (along with my own ticket):

You've come a long way, Baby,

And you're still going strong.

DAY 30 OF ABSTINENCE!

MARCH 1

English Class Journal
5:45–6:00 P.M.

I love my job as a television studio page. I realized this to a greater extent yesterday. After a week of car-induced absence, I couldn't wait to get back. Of course, a lot had to do with my renewed vitality. However, I really like what I do. Working at a television studio is exciting. It's fun. It's the right place for me to be now. The people, most of them at least, are so nice to be around. I feel like some of my energy comes through them.

It's true, at times, I was getting—I don't know, not bored, not tired—I'm not sure. Not totally thrilled with all the standing. Nothing, however, is totally thrilling all the time. At least, I don't think so. Nothing I have done so far has equaled the overall satisfaction (on a prolonged basis) I have felt at this. Seeing Perry on a consistent basis comes close, however. Well, it's a foot in the door. It's not stuck in there, though. It's just resting comfortably, tapping away to an invigorating beat.

BULIMICS TO RECEIVE HELP
BINGE/PURGE WHEN DISTRESSED

BY JANET SCHRIMMER

When the pressures of everyday life get to be too much for Cathy, she laces up her tennis shoes and takes a 30-minute jog. Andrea lights up another cigarette and Bill gets himself another beer.

Sharon has her own method of dealing with stress anxiety, she goes on an eating binge—devouring everything in sight, and then she forces herself to vomit it all out.

Sharon's behavior is a form of a disorder known as bulimia.

While bulimia has been around for years, the embarrassment felt by victims of the disorder has kept the problem hidden. The disorder is believed to affect tens of thousands of persons and is especially prevalent on college campuses among upper middle class women.

"The bulimic is usually a slender or normal weight woman who thinks she is overweight. Most tend to be attractive, well-groomed, and very high achievers. There is nothing physical about them that would make you think there was anything wrong with them," said Anita Siegman, a psychologist and director of University Counseling Services, who will be establishing a support group for bulimics at the university.

"Food temporarily relieves the anger and depression most of these women feel. When women haven't learned to deal effectively with either of these emotions, they may easily turn to food for a solution."

While daily patterns vary from bulimic to bulimic, the binge-purge obsessions are always present. Purging (to rid oneself) is usually done through vomiting, but extreme doses of laxatives are also commonly used.

"Most bulimics depend on their families very much, but they also strive to maintain independence. The need for perfection is often present, and that's why you see so many bulimics on college campuses. They're high achievers. They're obsessed with being thin and are often the classic 'good girls.'

"They often fear interpersonal intimacy—either on a sexual level or simply on a friendship level," Siegman said. Bulimics soon become so preoccupied with their binge-purge ritual that there's little time to develop or maintain relationships.

The purging following a binge relieves the guilt felt from overeating and prevents a weight gain. Eventually the urge becomes habit-forming and a lack of control is established. "This lack of control is the most frightening thing about the disorder, especially since most of these women have a lot of control in other areas of their life."

Most victims are between the ages of 18 to 25, however cases have been reported among women ages 13 to 60. The disease is extremely rare in men because the relentless pursuit of thinness is not so innate, Siegman said.

"This obsession to be thin has become more than a psychological problem. It has become a societal problem, especially here in California. Our society sends messages to women that tell them if they can't fit into a size-three jean then they haven't made it as a woman no matter what else they have going for them."

"The warmer weather of the West Coast and the additional recreational opportunities have also helped to create this preoccupation with the physical attractiveness of one's body. As a result there is a tremendous amount of pressure felt by women and many have a hard time accepting their bodies," Siegman said.

Siegman, who has counseled several women on an individual basis, plans to start a group, which will enable bulimics to share experiences and obtain help.

They often fear interpersonal intimacy . . .

Siegman and Eric Cohen, a Student Health Center physician, have directed several other groups and believe strongly in the notion that a group of-fers a tremendous amount of support and is a favorable method of obtaining therapy. It also helps participants view others who share a common problem and this helps banish feelings of isolation, Siegman said.

"The purpose of this group will be to assist women who feel caught in a cycle of binging and purging relative to eating behaviors. Specific techniques to control bulimia and to put food in perspective in one's total lifestyle will be dealt with in a safe and supportive atmosphere," Siegman said.

The group is scheduled to begin this week and is free of charge to students.

MARCH 1

"Point of No Return" Day 31

Well, I spoke with Anita Siegman, the University psychologist who's starting the groups today, and it looks like I'll be part of this very first eating disorder group at USC. I have to say, and I told her, I think I'm much better than I was. After all, as I told her, I haven't binged in over a month. Even though this group is popping up at a time when I'm coming out of it, it's the first time I might be able to talk to anyone, let alone people my own age, about this. Maybe I can even help people with my experiences. This, in addition to my weekly sessions with Francine, can only endorse what I've taught myself. I've been alone so long, I can't pass up an opportunity to finally talk.

MARCH 2

English Class Journal
11:35–11:50 A.M.

Written in car. While parked.

Writing as preventative medicine. Take it a minute at a time. Don't wonder what Bruce is thinking. Don't even think about the end of the evening until the end of the evening. You know you don't want to get involved romantically with this person. You're both pages at the television station, and you're friends.

You like him. Period. You want to stay friends. You will. This is not a date. This is just a day with a friend. Big deal. Enjoy it for what it is. Don't take it out of context or blow it out of proportion.

LATER: Well, yes, of course, he flirted with me, which, unlike some of the other pages, he has never done at work (maybe, because at six years older than me, he's more mature). He jokingly told me, "Oh, don't bat those huge brown eyes at me!" I think I looked so shocked at the comment, that he said, "Oh, come on, you must have hundreds of guys telling you what big, beautiful brown eyes you have!" But I just kept it very light and funny, and his flirts were as far as it went.

English Class Journal
12:05–12.20 P.M.

I defended Brent to Greg the other night. It was automatic. Of course, Greg was exceedingly paranoid about Brent's feelings toward him. Yet, I had nothing to gain, since Greg is the one I'm going out with, not Brent.

Brent, of course, does a better job as a TV studio page than Greg. In addition, he's a very interesting person. Quite nice looking in a sweet, pleasant way. The exterior exudes confidence and humor, but that is only part. He is not always sure of himself. That makes him all the more likeable. He will go far. He'll make it. He's got "it," that special something. Flair. Intelligence. Sincerity.

I like the guy. In fact, sometimes I wonder how much. I was flattered that such a desirable person fell for me. However, I did not want to be put in the position of losing Perry, and that's what it might have meant since it seemed like a relationship with Brent would have been a serious one.

I decided, though, that Brent's the second nicest boy (man? after all, he is 23, four years older than me) I've ever met. I always thought he put me on a pedestal, which was nice, but not the basis for a relationship. For those few non-platonic days it seemed different, like it could perhaps work. If it weren't for Perry, I would definitely go out with him.

MARCH 2

English Class Journal
6:30–6:45 P.M.

Well, I bypassed another one. It was not easy. At all. I could see myself eating the whole loaf of bread—in my mind. However, unlike the past, I didn't act on that mental image. I grabbed a diet soda instead.

I still "used" food. However, I added up calories, and decided what I would have beforehand. Eventually, I won't use food at all. I'm doing so much better. I'm really coming around. This was an accomplishment.

MARCH 3

"Point of No Return" Day 33

MARCH 4

"Point of No Return" Day 34

English Class Journal
1:55–2:10 P.M.

I'm sitting here in a television studio in the midst of a taping. A superstar is singing and after that will come four more. And I'm getting paid.

This is my dream job. Sometimes, it has become even blasé. But no, deep down and at all times a part of me realizes that this is fantastic. Whether I'm standing for hours, watching a light on a phone, or whatever, I do love it. Not just for the opportunities it offers and will offer, but because it's fun. The people are great. I'm making money. It's a sought-after position. Reflecting, I realized this is very long for me to stick to an optional activity. It's been eight months with never a thought of quitting.

I'm glad that I'm one of the young ones who will have the opportunity to work here for years.

MARCH 4

English Class Journal
2:10–2:25 P.M.

At Work.

Moving out by myself seems like the best thing to do. It will be exciting. New experiences always are. My own place. She, as a roommate, is intolerable. I'm not perfect, but she really goes too far, and probably doesn't even know it. But I don't want a roommate at all. It's not just her, although she epitomizes the pits of the pits.

I can't explain why I want to be alone; it's just a feeling. Maybe I won't like it. I think I will, and attitude is important.

There are, of course, advantages to living on campus, just as there are advantages to living with a roommate. There are disadvantages in each situation, too. All you can do is choose the situation that "seems" to have the most pluses and the least minuses. "Seems" is the operative word. You never know. But that's life, isn't it?

MARCH 4

English Class Journal
2:25–2:40 P.M.

At Work.

A DAY IN THE LIFE . . .

I woke up at 6:15 A.M. I had breakfast: 1 egg, 1 piece of French bread, 1 orange, 1 diet coffee milkshake. I made my bed. I exercised. I took a shower. I blew my hair dry. I got dressed. I wore jeans, a navy blue sweater with a preppy red shirt underneath. I wore my sandals, but one ripped and sent me flying in the garage. I got my stuff together. Put the water bottle out in the hall. Walked down the stairs. Had the shoe incident. Ran back up and changed shoes. Drove to school. Parked. Studied in library. Went to English Comp. at 9:30. Did Eng. exercises. Turned in journal. Ducked into library study carrel. Ate lunch there. Studied Spanish. Went to philosophy lecture on Plato's morality. Went to car. Had apple. Drove to work. Changed clothes. Went to stage six at the television studio. Was told to watch the phones.

MARCH 4

English Class Journal
3:30–3:45 P.M.
At Work.
Dear Perry,
This is a letter I'll never send because it tells the way I really feel. We never seem to tell each other that. I'm not complaining, at least that's why I'm not sending it. I don't want you to think that I'm complaining. I don't want to push you away. What I'd like is to be honest, and not have that honesty trigger any effects.

I guess what I really want to know (through mental telepathy, or some other painless method) is how you feel. Of course, this is my insecurity talking. I know that. That's another reason I'm not sending it. It's not a rational request. However, I still feel that way. I'm the type of person who doesn't like to feel I'm wasting my time (or energies), but you're worth wasting my time on, so I just won't ask.

MARCH 5

"Point of No Return" Day 35

MARCH 7

Well, I ate and I ruined it.
Like my life. I'm ruining my life.
God help me.

7. Momentary Hell

19 YEARS OLD

The absolute pits. I reached it today. I was totally unable to cope, to function. I never want to be here again.

I can't fit into my size-six page work uniform, except squeezed in, and it looks terrible. I've got to do something, foodwise, besides otherwise.

This is a many-faceted nightmare. I'm going to search through all this rubbish, straighten up a bit, and find myself among the ruins.

My first binge after a month of abstinence was a last-ditch effort to hold onto the past, a past that I saw disappearing. My focus has been askew for so long that I was afraid of seeing clearly.

I have so much strength and confidence. I try to make myself forget. I try to push it down. I try to create a false front of weakness, ugliness, and inability. The food serves as a hypnotic. Through it I begin to believe and live the false front. And yet, I know that my confidence and strength are locked away and being smothered. Why?

Part of my whole eating problem is that I have not been able to find a balance. I either do everything perfectly, or I do nothing, miserably. Why can't I just live somewhere in the middle? Why do I have to be at the extremes?

Before, losing weight equaled feeling good. Now, losing weight equals losing weight. Feeling good equals feeling good. The two are no longer inseparably linked. I am beginning to feel good about myself without any strings attached, i.e., the number on the scale or the amount or kind of food that goes into my body.

In reality, the real reason I should want to lose weight is to feel and look better. The number on the scale really does have nothing to do with that. It doesn't really represent anything.

"Point of No Return Re-Take" Days 36–41

DAILY TROJAN

OH, HOW I'LL MISS MY ROOMMATE'S BARBEQUED GRASSHOPPER CHILI

BY LISA MESSINGER

"Tushka poopkin farka!" Loosely translated this means, "Save room, we're having baked flies for dessert." Unfortunately, after finishing my moth-head and fish-eye casserole, I couldn't eat another bite.

But don't balk! Just a few short months ago, I, too, would have thought these delicacies unpalatable. However, my diet, as well as my lifestyle, has undergone radical changes since moving in with a foreign roommate.

Don't get me wrong. I'm by no means implying that living with a foreigner can't be a wonderfully enriching experience. And I'd be the first to jump at setting-up housekeeping with Hugh Grant or Antonio Banderas. It's just that my particular, isolated experience, while it may have been a thrill a minute, was a little too thrilling most of the time.

Of course, there were few benefits. I now know how to say "the toilet's backed-up" and "the dog ate the curtains" in two languages. But let's face it, after paying through the nose for rent, you expect more than a lesson in bilingual complaining.

Speaking of complaining, I didn't do any, I opted, instead for domestic tranquility. That was a mistake. I was driven to the point of raving resentment by not making known my dissatisfaction with my roommate's little idiosyncrasies. At first, I thought ours was just a cultural gap that could be bridged with a little patience and understanding. Believe me, I tried.

I accepted the fact that since animals are believed sacred in her country she couldn't be expected to remove the dog dropping/ sacrificial fur shrine that sat atop our kitchen table. Similarly, she couldn't be expected to shut the screens and deny entrance to what she called the "flying gods." Hard as it is to admit, when she wasn't busy praying to them, I secretly shot a few dozen with a squirt of Extra Strength Raid.

Since familial allegiance is next in importance to animal reverence, I couldn't expect her to ask her family to move the campsite they had set up in our living room. In fact, when they were inside the tent, I barely even noticed her four sisters, three brothers, mother, father, two cousins, great-grandmother and a man that, although no one seemed to know, could have been a distant relative.

Good sport that I am, I even submitted (at gun point) to a few family rituals. One night at the campfire, I was bequeathed to her brother. The wedding is set for early June. First, I have to spend three months in basic slave-training.

You're probably wondering, is there no end to my patience? Yes, there is an end. I *can* tolerate almost anything. However, there are some acts so inconsiderate, so irritating, that no apartment co-renter should be forced to put up with. My month's notice has been given because of such an act. You guessed it—she blocked my parking space with her Porsche. Let's face it— there's only so much I can take. I do have to admit, however, I'm going to miss that barbequed grasshopper chili that only she could make.

Lisa Messinger is a freshman majoring in journalism.

Dear Perry,

I was *going* to lie. I was all set to lie. But then I realized that although it's relatively easy for me to lie to other people, I just don't want to lie to you. It would be easier (and from outside appearances more acceptable) to give an excuse (e.g., "I am deathly ill," which is what I was going to say) than it is to even try to give a truthful explanation. However, I'm tired of giving excuses and lying (not to you, just in general.) So, I decided to be honest, especially with someone I love. Yes, I admit it. I love you. (I didn't say I was *in* love with you. There's only so much I can reveal.)

I'm not here. I tried to call you at home and dorm to lie about ruining tonight, but maybe this will be better in the long run. At least I feel like a lead weight is being lifted from my chest. You see, I have been living a double life, like two people. I guess I just can't take it anymore. I don't know why else I would be writing this now. I have and have had (for eleven years) a problem. It is only recently that I have begun to come to grips with it. And I *am* getting much better.

(Now is the time to read the articles I enclosed, they explain it as well as and less emotionally than I could.)

BULIMIA: THE BINGING/PURGING DILEMMA

By Francine Snyder

Bulimia . . . what is it? Like anorexia nervosa, it is an eating disorder affecting thousands of people. And it is finally out of the bathroom.

Have you heard of impulsive or binge eating? Bulimia is characterized by the consumption of large quantities of food. Whole cakes, gallons of ice cream, bags of cookies are often consumed along with large quantities of liquid. Purging follows, and is usually brought about by forced vomiting. Sometimes diuretics and laxatives are used, and sometimes the "purge" is through compulsive exercise or starvation dieting.

The following are typical comments from clients while in the middle of a binge: "I know I am hurting myself, but I don't care." "I don't care if I get cancer from doing this." "I don't care if I die, I just have to get rid of all this food I ate . . . In fact, I wish I were dead." "I can't stand doing this any longer and I can't stand not to do this. The thought of

giving it up is just too much for me to bear."

Most bulimics learn about vomiting from a parent, friend, or relative who has tried the same behavior. The eating and vomiting start out as a lark—it is a way for an individual to literally have her cake and eat it, too.

The bulimic is generally female and the binging/purging begins sometime around adolescence. It is usually during adolescence that a girl experiences her first rejection. Binging and purging initially solves two problems: It allows her to eat whatever she wants without having to suffer the consequences of a weight gain. And stuffing the food is a great way of avoiding any feelings of anger, hurt, or rejection she may be experiencing. Vomiting or other purging relieves the stuffed, bloated, uncomfortable feeling the overeating brings about. The behavior becomes obsessive; there is almost nothing that will stop a bulimic individual from binging.

The cycle is addictive and causes an extreme amount of shame, guilt, isolation, and fear of getting caught.

Men are affected by this disorder but to a lesser degree than women. They usually chance upon it after losing weight, when they are besieged with the fear of regaining what they have lost. The binging allows the man to eat whatever he wants and the vomiting enables him to maintain his present weight. In general, there is less social and parental pressure on the male to be "thin." A man is allowed to have more bulk.

For the bulimic living alone, the likelihood of someone coming home unexpectedly is not a problem. However, for someone in a relationship or with children, there is the constant fear of getting caught. Imagine the mortification of having just completed a secret binge of a chocolate cake, a half-gallon of vanilla ice cream, and a bag of cookies. There you sit amidst empty cartons, torn bags, and containers of food, and in walks your spouse. What do you do? What can you say?

Ah, what a relief when you put your children to bed. You are finally alone and can eat and vomit without any distractions. But what happens if the children wake up? Yes, you can tell them you are sick, but how many times can you use that as an excuse?

Noise from the shower may appear to be a great camouflage technique, but what happens when it backfires? What if it wakes someone up, how do you explain running the shower at 2 A.M.?

Then there is the problem of dates and appointments and getting places on time. You leave the office at 5:30 P.M., you make a stop at the supermarket on the way home. You load up with ice cream, cake, crackers, doughnuts, and whipped cream—and a sandwich so you will have something to eat in the car on the way home. You'd love some peanuts or peanut butter, but you know that those foods are too difficult to bring up. As you check out, you make some remark to the cashier about the party you are giving, because you would just die if anyone found out about your secret life and that all that food is for you. Then you are off, tearing into the

sandwich as you get into the car and mumbling to yourself how it's OK to eat the sandwich because you haven't eaten all day.

It's all very exciting and lots of fun. You can eat whatever you want, all those foods you would never allow yourself to eat before because you were always on a diet. Besides, you are extremely health conscious; "Sugar, who me? I never eat sugar. I'm strictly into health foods, fruits, vegetables, tofu. I practice yoga twice a week and work out at the gym at least three times a week." And, after all, your friends know how "good" you are. They always tell you how envious they are that you are able to resist the hot fudge sundaes and fresh-baked cookies and stay so thin. They all wonder how you can have such incredible willpower. God, what if any of your friends caught you loading up on all this junk food? How would you explain yourself? Oh well, don't worry about that now. You've got your sandwich, doughnuts, and cookies; you're OK.

The bulimic is usually able to function well at work and is often in a top-level executive position. An outsider viewing the typical bulimic would probably say the individual has everything she could possibly want. She is likely to have a good figure (average weight or thinner), earn a good salary, have a lot of people around, and be extremely competent at her work. She is the kind of person that you admire, respect, and perhaps envy.

But there is another side; a side no one sees. The part that is constantly obsessed with food from the moment she wakes up until she falls asleep at night. A great many binge eaters will wake up during the night to eat.

A sample entry in the bulimic's journal might read as follows: I get home almost running in the door and stop only long enough to put the grocery bag down. I go over to pull the phone out of the wall while munching on a doughnut. The last thing I want is for the phone to ring. Ah, peace and quiet and tranquility. It's just me and the food. How wonderful! No hassles, no aggravation. No one to bug me. Just peace and quiet and food. What fun!

One hour later—UGH! My stomach is so

bloated I can hardly breathe. Ugh, I'd better drink some more water to make sure I will get up all the food. I'd better vomit now. If I wait too long, I won't be able to get it all out. Ugh, I can hardly make it to the bathroom. I'm so uncomfortable. My stomach is so bloated. I can't move. This is awful. I can't wait to get some relief, to feel the rush of food as it comes up.

Oh, what a mess, how disgusting. God, I wish I could stop this binge eating. I put my finger down my throat again. What if my friends or business associates saw me now. Vice-president of a thriving company. What a joke! I feel like a two-headed freak — a Dr. Jekyll/Mr. Hyde. Well, I can't think about it now. I have to concentrate on getting up all the food I ate. Good thing I ate that vanilla ice cream — it comes up so easily.

What time is it? My gosh, it's 7 P.M. I have a date at 8 P.M. I still have to finish vomiting, clean up the bathroom, shower, and get dressed. I hope I can make it on time. I've got to keep this up until I've gotten rid of every bit of food I ate and my stomach is completely flat again. Hope my puffy eyes don't give

me away. Oh well, John probably won't notice. I hope he won't notice the swollen glands in my neck. I wonder if they would go away if I would stop binging. If only I could stop.

The binging and vomiting is an endless struggle. Once backed into this behavior, it is extremely difficult to break the pattern. Some form of counseling or psychotherapy is required to treat the cause, assist in changing the patterns, and to teach techniques that will break the binging/purging behavior. Support and encouragement are needed for the bulimic who has an addiction that is often as entrenched as the addiction to drugs or alcohol.

As a therapist, I view this condition as an opportunity; as a beginning, not an end. It is a time when the individual can turn what has been a negative behavior into a positive learning experience. The food and eating can be viewed in a positive light when it is used symbolically as an aid to the therapeutic process.

Therapy is important to help the clients recognize their needs and learn how to fulfill those needs in a more rewarding manner.

So, Perry, now you know. I don't want you to feel sorry for me. There's no need. Most of the time (some of the time, at least) I'm a pretty confident, "together" person. Francine Snyder, the woman in the article, has been helping me to help myself, as one of the people she described who binges and then purges through compulsive exercise and starvation dieting. And I have been. Just writing this is helping me (it's a big step), and I thank you for being someone I could write it to. So why couldn't I see you? Part of this condition is that we have rules we make ourselves live by. Rules for *everything*. My biggest rule has been that if I don't follow all the rules, I cannot see anyone that I want to see. Honestly, I feel like there is no way I could face you (I was literally panicking). I have broken more dates—I hardly will ever let myself see my friends—I've been lonely.

I'm in the process of changing this, but I'm not totally ready yet. And I want to see you. You said on the phone when we were planning our date that you missed me. I missed you a lot, but I'm just not ready yet. When I was going to lie about this weekend, I was going to say I could see you next week (but I knew I probably wouldn't feel right about it yet). I do want to see you very much, but I feel like I'd like to wait a few weeks. I can handle the phone, though. I'm not putting pressure on you to call me, and will understand if you don't. To be honest, after this, I'll be scared when I talk to you.

Sometimes I feel envious of you. You seem so well-adjusted, so happy with yourself and your body image, with school, etc. In important ways, you're much less inhibited than I am, and I'd like to be more like that.

Deep inside I do have a lot of faith in myself, my abilities, and my worthiness. It's just that up until now I have put a lot of my energy (and I have a lot of energy) into squelching the confidence and strength that I have. Now that I've realized this, I'm trying to figure out why and change it. A while ago, I would never have been able to write this. I would have felt as if I was exposing my whole self and identity, and if it were rejected or misunderstood so would I be. Now, I have it more in perspective. This is only one part of me. It's not all of me. It's not my whole life. I've changed, but I'm still me. And I'm not afraid anymore. I do love you, and it feels good to say it. For me, it doesn't mean anything has to happen, change anything, or imply anything. It's just the way I feel.

P.S. Just to keep this honesty bit up, after I decided to write this, I unplugged my phone just in case you got my message. I knew it was important for me to write this, and I thank you for being someone I could write it to. I'd have chickened out if I had talked to you. Please excuse my seemingly strange behavior. But even if you don't, I know it was better for me than lying.

P.P.S. I'll be at my parents' home from now on.

MARCH 30

Perry: What did she want?!

Joey: To talk to you.

Perry: What about?

Joey: I don't know. I'm your brother, not your answering service! We talked for a half hour. You didn't come up much.

Perry: That's encouraging, Joey. Why didn't you tell me yesterday?

Joey: It slipped my mind.

Perry: Terrific, just great. We've got a date tonight, and I want to know why she called! It might be important.

Joey: So call her, Dipshit.

Perry: Yea, I just might do that.

Hmmm. . . no answer. Well, I'm probably worrying about nothing. If it was really important she would have called again. But still . . .

From that moment on a bad feeling overtook my mind and body. A feeling somewhere between anxiety and nausea. A feeling that I tried to get rid of but failed. Two o'clock call, no answer; three, no answer; four, no answer; five, no answer; five thirty, I wanted to call, but I was afraid, afraid that you might have been home, and you would've thought it was strange that I was worried that you might not be able to go out. And I was afraid that you wouldn't be there to answer, and I would know for sure you weren't going out with me. So, I didn't call. I went in the shower, blow-dried my hair, brushed my teeth, got dressed, finalized my plans for the evening, drove to the gas station, and then, finally, I arrived at your apartment at seven thirty on the dot.

The idea that you would stand me up seemed completely ridiculous, at least that's what I told myself.

"She wouldn't do that tonight. We've been planning this night for weeks. It's just impossible." So, in that frame of mind, but still that nagging feeling underlining my confident talk, I jumped out of the car and ran up the steps all set to press #207.

"Oh shit! What's this 'Perry Schwartz' thing?" I tore open the envelope, read the first two pages of your letter, and quickly decided that I had better retreat to the safe confines of the car before I did something rash, like screaming.

There it all was in black and white and Xerox, and I could scarcely believe it was true. I kept looking up at your balcony half hoping I would catch you smiling as if this were some elaborate practical joke. But this was no joke. My fears had been confirmed, and I had the sensation of being almost, well, relieved.

Why should I feel relieved? I asked myself. For one thing, all the tension that I had built up in anticipation of the evening had been released (although not in the way I should have liked!!!). And, moreover, you not being there freed me to do other things. (Like dine at a fast-food restaurant and take in a film by myself.) But there was one problem: Your problem. If it was hard for me to believe that you weren't there, it was even harder for me your reason why!

It all seemed so fantastic.

BULIMIA. The infamous Roman technique of gluttony. I could not understand how you could consider yourself a bulimic. I don't think you are. You don't purge yourself by vomiting, so you aren't really. Did you really eat junk food secretly and in vast amounts? I can't envision it! But it would certainly go some way in explaining your meager eating habits that I have seen. When did you come to the conclusion that you were a bulimic and how? Why did it make you develop a rule that never existed before? I am really confused. Do you have to punish yourself to improve? It doesn't seem reasonable.

Another thing you wrote disturbed me. You should not envy me or anyone else. Just as you appear very "together" but have problems, so do we all. I am sure I have just as many personality and confidence difficulties as you. For example, every time I develop the notion that I am good, great, studly, cute, nice, smart, handsome, or just okay, I immediately tell myself I'm a jerk and an asshole (sometimes too loudly!). This is just my way of keeping my ego in check and improving myself. So, you see, I'm not always the confident, self-assured individual you seem to think I am. In fact, my way of controlling my ego frequently succeeds so well as to make me fear risking anything that might be personally embarrassing. (Why do you think I never asked you out on a date before you asked me?!) You should not envy anyone, least of all *this* jerk writing this.

Lisa, if what you wrote is true, and I have my doubts, I wish that you will succeed in correcting your problem straight away. I want to see you and talk to you (but the phone is too much for me this week). I am still numb from Saturday night. The movies by yourself, and making up stories about what you did the night before, is not my idea of fun. I had and still have other ideas, ideas that include I hope, *you.*
Soon, I hope.

Love,
Perry

Why Self-Treatment Doesn't Work

At this point Lisa is only too painfully aware that her eating disorder has begun to spin wildly out of control with dire consequences, and yet a part of her still believes that self-help is the answer. You probably know just where Lisa is. You may be confused, scared, lonely, and depressed but you still feel you can regain control. You are strong and independent and have always been able to handle anything in the past. Just another diet, increased exercise, another journal, and more self-promises. Try a little harder, control your thoughts, and change your attitude. Perhaps a new boyfriend, a move, or a job change. Then there are a few days, a month or even a few months of abstinence— healthy eating, no binging and purging. You will think that you are home free and feel wonderful. You have regained control . . . or have you?

Unfortunately, you are finding that it is just not that simple. These chapters follow the important limbo or white knuckling period, a time when you are somewhat aware that what you are doing is not working in the way you expected. At the same time a part of you still believes that self-help is the answer. A part of your mind is now saying this is no good; this is extremely dangerous. I have lost control. My life is falling apart. I don't want to be caught up in this cycle anymore. An equally strong part of your mind is saying this may have happened to Lisa but it won't happen to me. I can outsmart it. I know what I am doing and what will happen. This can not and will not bring me down. Others may have succumbed but I will not! Even though you know something is vitally wrong, you still think you can handle it yourself, in effect that you can fix it, and you try and try and try. There may be good periods followed by relapse and sinking into old patterns, then control and another "good" period followed by relapse. This is the myth of self-help. No matter how strong a person you are, this situation is different. As much as your mind tells you that you can help yourself, in reality you just can't, because you have still not addressed what this is really all about.

In this chapter I will look, with you, at some of the issues that begin to emerge during this important time. I will begin by looking at the issue of control. If you are like Lisa, at this point you may be feeling very out of control. Your world, as you have known it, may seem upside-down. Things around you are changing and frequently not at all the way you expected. The question of identity and "who am I" may reemerge.

We will look at relationships because, again, you, like Lisa, may seek to regain control and find some of these answers in relationships, particularly relationships with boyfriends. We know that at this time you are still insecure about reaching out and may have little real trust in relationships at all, let alone their ability to be of any real help. Perhaps most importantly we will look at guilt, shame, and secrets because it is during this limbo period that you will begin to come face to face with the "lie," the secret life you have been living to maintain your eating disorder and your façade.

This limbo period is a very difficult and painful time, in part because many of you continue the struggle alone. It is also a hopeful time when new insights and important growth begins. Most importantly it is the time when you realize that self-help alone is not working and that you cannot do it alone. You must seek professional help. You will find that your new strength lies in reaching out.

Lisa did seek professional help, although the road, as we will see in the next chapters, was not always a smooth one. Some people with eating disorders continue to believe that self-help alone is the answer, and may stay in this limbo period for a very long time, sometimes as much as decades. The road to recovery can be a long and difficult one but at some point there must be a beginning. The first step is the hardest, and even though reaching out may be the hardest thing you have ever done, no one can make this journey alone.

I am aware that many of you are reading Lisa's story because you share her journey. Others of you have a friend or loved one with an eating disorder. When I give lectures I always hear the question: "I have a friend or family member with an eating disorder. How can I help them?" It is essential to realize that without help the eating disorder will only become worse. Lisa made the decision to seek help on her own. This is frequently not the case. I have far too often seen eating disorders progress to a life-threatening stage with the patient either unaware of the severity of what is happening or unwilling or unable to reach out for help. It is at this point that you must intervene. For different reasons many of my patients come for help only at the urging or insistence of a friend or family member. It is to you, the friend or family member, that I address the all-important last part of this chapter. Self-help is not possible. Professional help for someone you care about may mean the difference between life and death.

Lisa finds herself on a rapidly spiraling downward curve. Let's move back to her story in the hopes that Lisa's dilemma, her attempts at resolution, and her final decision to seek help will provide valuable insights for you in your own quest for understanding.

SEEKING CONTROL

In the limbo chapter, Lisa finds herself struggling with issues of control, structure, and identity, and in a position she would never have imagined. Lisa, the straight-A student who could do anything, could not make it through her first semester of college and has come home. Maintaining a perfect face to the world had always been important, and although Lisa does not talk about it in her diary, we can only imagine what facing her friends, and in particular her father, meant to her and how awful it must have been.

For most of my clients this limbo time is not only depressing and frightening, but also very confusing. They are trying desperately to make sense out of what is happening to them. Lisa writes on November 8: "What's in store for me? Can I control it? Why did I leave school midterm? The reasons, I have a feeling, are more complex than I seem to be experiencing. Do I still love myself? Where's the feeling of ecstasy that I had in the summer when I first lost the weight? I want it back. I've got to try. I may have answers, but I can't give up. No matter what, I'm going to do it. Confidence. That's what I need. I can and will help myself. Ecstasy, here I come."

This paragraph summarizes much of what I hear from my clients, and it will probably sound very familiar to you. You feel out of control. You are confused. You really do not understand what is happening to you. You are failing at things that would have seemed so easy in the past. You long for the initial feeling of euphoria that you felt with the first big weight loss. You still do not understand that the euphoria was an illusion and will never return in quite the same way, although at this stage weight losses still do have a powerful impact on mood regulation. You are only beginning to perceive that what is happening to you has only partially to do with body size and weight and even more to do with intimacy, identity, structure, and control. You may still firmly believe you can pull it all together and get yourself out of what is happening to you alone. You still believe self-help is the answer. At this point only one thing remains clear—you do not want to gain weight.

As we read Lisa's November 8 entry, we feel hopeful that Lisa has begun to see the larger picture, but that is not yet the case. On November 10, only two days later, she returns again to obsessive charting of food and weight and states, "This is the most important thing in my life." Lisa, at this moment, is primarily aware that she has begun to lose control. Other insights are more peripheral. She quickly returns to tried and true mechanisms to regain control, losing weight. Lisa returns to food and exercise charting, and as we will soon see, relationships. For most of my clients, this period is one of beginning insights and quick return to the eating disorder. Why, we might ask, is this the case? A move forward and then a slip back. Let's try to understand a little better what is happening.

Control

We have already talked about control as a central component in an eating disorder. For all of my patients, the body serves as a metaphor. If they can control their body, they can control the world around them. As they begin to gain insights, they will lose some of these controls, and that is terrifying. "Cure" becomes a fearful prospect. Their eating disorder has been their lifeline. For some it has been their only friend as their self-imposed isolation increased. Through each crisis the eating disorder has been there as the sole friend who offers comfort and understands. It has also served as a force supporting the need for control. In a time of enormous confusion it continues to help you create what appears to be a more stable structure, even though none of the above is in reality true. The most important part is that you are only beginning to realize that this best friend is your worst enemy. This enemy has completely taken over control and, on some level, you know that it has the power to completely destroy your mind and your body. However, for now, these thoughts are still not completely clear. At this point, most will begin to do anything they can to regain control, firmly believing that if they can only regain control (at this point over their body) all will return to normal (whatever normal is believed to be). And so over and over, as there seems to be progress, the eating disorder continues to regain control.

In addition, the ongoing struggle between dependence and independence is a key one and most believe they must and can regain these controls entirely on their own. After all, many have always been able to do almost anything on their own, and like Lisa, at this point still believe they CAN regain control. In addition, seeking help means turning over some of their control to others. That is also a frightening prospect. Thus, the struggle, for now, remains a private and lonely one.

Structure and Identity

Deeply entwined with control is the struggle for structure and identity. Lisa writes: "My first binge after a month of abstinence was a last-ditch effort to hold onto the past, a past that I saw disappearing. My focus has been askew for so long that I was afraid of seeing clearly. I have so much strength and confidence. I try to make myself forget. I try to push it down. I try to create a false front of weakness, ugliness, and inability. The food serves as a hypnotic. Through it I begin to believe and live the false front. And yet I know that my confidence and strength are locked away and being smothered. Why?"

The answer to this "why" lies in part in the following paragraph: "I remember reading about how a former fatty must mourn for her "fat self," someone she has had such an intensive love-hate relationship with for so long. I also remember thinking that this did not apply to me. That was then; this is now. I believe I am grieving. It has begun to hit me that the old me is gone, really gone. I don't know where she is. She must be dead. A big part of me has died. Although, for the most part, I didn't like this person, I cared about her. Not liking yourself is misery, but it becomes routine and almost comfortable. Not knowing yourself, however, is scary as hell."

Another component in an eating disorder has to do with developmental delays in the formation of identity. Later, Lisa writes to Perry that although she was not initially aware of it, her preoccupation with food and weight had been going on for eleven years—key years in the formation of adult identity. When Lisa entered college she consciously knew she wanted to become a different person. Again her weight and body size became the metaphor—that person that she wanted to be was a thin person. She wanted to leave behind her "old fat self" and with it so many of the complex parts of her identity that had begun to form during her high school years. She believed that if she lost weight, she would be different. This created a huge and scary void. If she was no longer the person she was in high school, who was she?

To fill the void Lisa created (or certainly intensified the already existing) complex superstructure centering on body size and weight that has formed the core of her eating disorder. Her eating disorder is the known. Everything else is unknown. She is her eating disorder; they are one and the same. Giving up her eating disorder would mean giving up her fragilely formed identity, giving up herself. She cannot let that happen. She cannot go for help. That would mean losing herself, because for right now her eating disorder is all she has, and what, on some level, holds her together. This is key!

RELATIONSHIPS

You may have found that another way of maintaining control, structure, and identity is through relationships—primarily through relationships with boyfriends. Even during this confusing period, having a boyfriend makes Lisa feel more whole and in control. A boyfriend also seems to provide a clearer sense of her rapidly faltering identity. As long as we have known Lisa, this pattern has been true. From the first pages of her diary we see Lisa trying to be what she imagines the current boyfriend wants her to be, gaining a part of her identity from the current boyfriend. A relationship means not only identity but also control.

All of Lisa's relationships seem to have two things in common. First, the superficial appearance—all of the men are good looking, charming, and popular. These are the men Lisa seeks to enhance her own identity and sense of self. Second, although we are aware of their outward appearances, we know little about who these men really are, how they think, feel, and react. Despite ongoing entries about Perry, we also know very little about who he is. At the same time, we are continuously surprised that none of them, including Perry, have any idea of the real Lisa, and of her secret life. During this limbo stage, relationships with boyfriends are not the only problem. Lisa has begun to isolate and we hear nothing about girlfriends either. As the controls unravel it becomes harder and harder to maintain the same façade. Some of my patients are able to do it, but many, like Lisa, find it easier to retreat and isolate. For most, even the closest friends and family members have little idea of the extent of the illness. Lisa ostensibly leaves her roommate because of the roommate's bad habits, but as most of you know, it is easier to pursue your eating disorder in isolation. As the eating disorder progresses, the isolation increases.

As we look at relationships, it is essential to look at your relationship with food. For a long time your eating disorder has been your primary relationship. Unlike other relationships in your life, whenever you have needed it, the eating disorder has always been there. During periods of stress, confusion, and pain, food and your eating disorder have provided comfort and numbing. Your restrained eating, exercise routine, and binging or purging are all known, and seem under control at times in your life when other things feel confusing and out of control. On so many levels your eating disorder is or was your best friend. However, this is a friendship with an often unexpected and terrible price. Again, you are becoming increasingly aware that this best friend has become your worst enemy.

GUILT, SHAME, AND SECRETS

It is important to note here that all eating disorders don't follow exactly the same pattern. Some of Lisa's issues will feel very true and real for you, while in other cases you will find yourself saying, "That's just not me, maybe I really don't have a problem." Please do not draw that conclusion just because your experience differs from Lisa's. It is important to remember that Lisa's eating disorder may, in some ways, be different from yours and cannot be clearly defined or labeled. The following elements of guilt, shame, and secrecy are what I see in some of my patients, and can serve as a further guide—but again, should not be taken as absolutes. There are many similarities to the various kinds of eating disorders, but also some real differences. In the next paragraphs I will make some brief distinctions.

One important distinction lies in what keeps patients from seeking help. Patients come for treatment when their coping mechanisms no longer work. Many of my anorectic patients believe that their coping mechanisms are working; they are getting thinner and thinner, so why should they need help? Remember the patient I described in *Getting Thin Is Not the Answer*? She truly believed she was fine and beautiful as her body weight dropped below 80 pounds. Only when she could not climb steps or even get out of bed without difficulty and when others were staring at her did she begin to think she had a problem. Even then, at this life-threatening stage, it took the intervention of others to get her help. In terms of guilt, there usually is none for anorectics; after all, they are thin and thin is good. Shame about their bodies may have to do with past trauma, sexual abuse, or family of origin dynamics but usually has little to do with their current diet and body weight, although they rarely allow others to see them unclothed. Again, thinner is better, their mechanisms for achieving that thinness are certainly completely intact, and until a dangerous point is reached they are often not consciously aware that what they are doing is really putting their life in danger.

For many of my bulimic patients, as with my clients with binge eating disorder, something else is occurring that makes secrecy even more essential. Bulimics see their binging and purging as disgusting and shameful, even though what they are really dealing with is a highly addictive cycle that is very difficult to break. They constantly wonder what others would think about them if they only knew. They are fully aware that the face they present to the world is often diametrically opposed to what they feel like inside, and that it is essential to maintain the façade.

All of this contributes to strong feelings of self-loathing, which may be accompanied by massive guilt at the lie they are living. As the disease progresses this lie becomes harder and harder to maintain. Finally it becomes impossible to continue the lie. Lisa writes to Perry, "I was going to lie. I was all set to lie. . . . However, I'm tired of giving excuses and lying (not to you, just in general). . . . I have and have had (for eleven years) a problem." Only when the veil of secrecy begins to lift can cure begin.

For all of my eating-disordered clients, secrecy is key, as they find themselves caught more and more in a growing web of deceit and lies. One of the ways of maintaining the lie is to increase isolation. It is impossible to consume very large quantities of food in the presence of others. In fact, when most of my patients are in social situations, eating is often restrained. Having a roommate makes secrecy and binge eating and purging more difficult. Thus, Lisa cites many problems with her roommate, but we are left to wonder if some of these problems are rationalizations to enable Lisa to leave the roommate and live alone and continue her double life more easily. In any case, increasing isolation is essential as the lie, with its concomitant guilt and shame, progresses.

Because of the guilt, shame, and secrecy, coming to another person for help and self-revealing is a monumental task, even though the person to whom the eating-disordered individual turns is usually empathetic, concerned, caring, and not judgmental. In addition, when my bulimic patients come for help, what they are sometimes initially seeking is a "cure" to stop the binge and purge behavior. Nothing more. They know that they have gone beyond the "point of no return." Only later do the real treatment goals emerge.

"No One Can Help Me"

Although in Lisa's case it is unclear what part clinical depression played in the development of her eating disorder, it is clear that Lisa is now very depressed. She sees her life unraveling, her eating disorder spinning wildly out of control, and is aware that in her need for secrecy she has cut off everyone who can help her. In addition, one of the primary indicators of clinical depression is the sense that there is no light at the end of the tunnel. There is not only the feeling that you are out of control and can no longer change things, but also the feeling that things cannot and will not ever change. **That is not true.** Although, for now, as these feelings cycle, there are long periods when hope is lost. Even though you are now aware that self-help is not working, you may also feel, like Lisa, totally alone. You may feel that no one could ever understand what you are experiencing. You may feel sure that no one can help. You are wrong! It is important to realize that at this point it may be your depression that is speaking. There is help and someone who will understand and help you begin the long road to recovery.

BEGINNING INSIGHTS

There is indeed a light at the end of the tunnel for Lisa, as there will be for you, and we begin to see that light in these chapters. As Lisa's controls begin to break down, we are witnessing the beginning of some important insights that will become essential to her later recovery. You, too, will find that insights begin to emerge, but may be quickly pushed back under by fears of change and a move back to the safety and "security" of your disorder. In the beginning this is a normal process and it is important to not be discouraged. As Lisa has said over and over, "It is a slippery path." You are just beginning your road to recovery. Keep going. Perhaps some of the following will sound familiar to you.

Finding a Balance

A brief note on perfectionism bears mentioning. For the first time, Lisa gains some insights into her need to be the perfect person. She writes: "Part of my whole eating problem is that I have not been able to find a balance. I either do everything perfectly or I do nothing, miserably. Why can't I just live somewhere in the middle? Why do I have to be at the extremes?"

In the midst of an eating disorder, balance is impossible. As I have mentioned, for a person with an eating disorder, everything is black or white. Perfect is white. All else is black. From weight, to foods, to body size, to exercise, to relationships, in fact to everything in the world around you, imperfect is considered "bad." Purely and simply, perfection is just not possible. Finding a balance and appreciating the shades of gray is essential to cure. As you get better you will find your balance and, like Lisa, will be amazed at how much easier life can be.

Looking Inside, Not Outside

Lisa has begun to, more and more, look inside for the answers. She writes, "It wasn't until I turned eighteen, attended college, and fell in love that I realized the absurdity of my attitude. No outside event can cause a lasting significant change. We can't depend on others or outside events to make us happy. These can only enhance an already fulfilled individual. They do not create one." Initially these realizations remain intellectualized and are not as yet integrated, but the journey is beginning. As in all other areas, initial insight is quickly followed by a slide back into old patterns, and the same evening Lisa writes again about her idealized love for Perry, stating, "I yearn for the security that will make me feel secure in my insecurity." She is increasingly aware of her insecurity but she feels the solution still lies in a relationship and not in herself.

Separating Food From Your Identity

Lisa is beginning to separate who she is from what she eats and her body weight. She writes, "My first binge after a month of abstinence was a last ditch effort to hold on to the past, a past that I saw disappearing. My focus has been askew for so long that I was afraid of seeing clearly. . . . Before, losing weight equaled feeling good. Now, losing weight equals losing weight. Feeling good equals feeling good. The two are no longer inseparably linked. I am beginning to feel good about myself without any strings attached, i.e., the number on the scale or the amount and kind of food that goes into my body."

In the past, all of Lisa's emotions—sad, happy, fearful, and confused, as well as her successes and failures—were in direct relation to her eating disorder. This is beginning to change. Throughout these chapters she is becoming aware that who she is consists of more than just her body weight. She is also gaining initial insight into the fact that thin does not necessarily mean happy.

A GUIDE FOR FAMILY AND FRIENDS

Lisa has finally reached the point where she is realizing that self-help does not work. She has contacted a psychologist for individual therapy and will also begin group therapy. As of yet we know little about this process. We are also not fully aware of the part Lisa's mother has played in her decision to get help. For all practical purposes the decision seems to have been Lisa's, although speaking to her new counselor and then Perry seems to have opened the floodgates.

For some eating-disordered individuals this is simply not the case. It is not unusual for many people with an eating disorder to not seek outside help on their own. For these individuals their eating disorder is like an addiction to alcohol or drugs, and as long as it seems to be working, and for all the above reasons I have discussed, they do not want, or are really unable at this time to seek help. That's where family and friends can step in. Many of my patients enter treatment reluctantly and only at the persistent urging or sometimes demands and ultimatums of family or friends. This can be a difficult and tricky process. Although you may have long suspected your loved one or friend has an eating disorder, you may not have been sure. In most cases you have not had any idea how to intervene. Hopefully the following tips can be of help to you in approaching your loved one.

Learn About Eating Disorders

Begin by learning all that you can about eating disorders. You have made a good start by reading this book. Books, articles, and brochures are everywhere. The Internet is an excellent source of information. ANRED (Anorexia Nervosa and Related Eating Disorders, Inc.) and EDAP (Eating Disorders Awareness and Prevention) are among the many sources that provide practical and very useful information. (See the Resource List on page 237 for a comprehensive list.) Most states have eating-disorder professional organizations, and the national and international organizations like IADEP (International Association of Eating Disorder Professionals) provide a wealth of available information. A professional is frequently available by phone, email, or fax to answer specific questions. Don't be afraid to ask! Even if hospitalization is not an issue, eating-disorder hospital programs across the country are only too happy to send out brochures and very helpful general information.

It is important to begin to know the difference between facts and myths about weight, body size, food, nutrition, and exercise. This information will help you to understand some of the complexity and difficulty that your friend or loved one is going through. It may also help you to understand the extent of their pain. Knowing these facts may help you confront some of their illusions and inaccuracies when the time is right. As we are well aware of with Lisa, the process is a slow one, and the time may not be right quite yet for confrontations about truth and facts. Be patient. However, try to ascertain whether the situation is life-threatening and demands immediate action. If not . . .

Make the Approach

Wherever I speak to groups, the question of how to approach a friend comes up. It is a difficult problem. Confronting your friend or family member will be not be easy and you may find that you want to put it off. At first you may not be sure that what you have perceived is real. You may feel that bringing up this issue, which to date has been a finely guarded secret, may jeopardize your relationship. In some cases you will be right. In other cases your friend will be relieved to have someone to talk to and to know that you care. What is most important to remember is that your friend, no matter what the face to the world, is suffering. This can be a matter of life and death. As far as we know, early on, no one confronted Lisa, and so for eleven years her disease ran its deadly course. Sometimes early intervention and confrontation can make all of the difference.

Choose a quiet, private, and unrushed time and place to talk. Approach your friend or family member with love, caring, and most of all respect. She is going through hell and you must respect how difficult it is for her to talk about or even admit what is occurring. Be caring, but firm. Do not be manipulated. Remember that your friend has been used to pretending and lying. Again respect that the truth is difficult and painful. If your friend is willing to talk, listen and listen and listen. Try not to give advice at least initially, as it will often not be taken. All of the things you want to say are probably things your friend has thought about before. Talk to your friend about what you have seen and what you have found out about eating disorders. Be kind and try to be brief. There will be so much you want to say, because you care so much about the person, but there will be time later. Do not shame, nag, or reinforce guilt. Try to talk only minimally about weight and size. Emphasize health and recovery. Emphasize hope. Let the person know that you will be there to help.

Reinforce the Need for Professional Help

You are there to help your friend or family member better find her way. Hear her pain and reinforce that help is possible and there is a better way. At this point your primary task is love, support, caring, and hope. You are not a professional and this is just an opening. If possible, use this opening to get your friend or family member professional help. This may not be easy, but the feeling that you can do the job alone is just another illusion and may do more damage than good. No matter how much you love the person and how strong you are, professional help is the only door out of this deadly disease.

The other scenario I frequently hear is this: "What if my friend or family member refuses to talk about it and says it just isn't true or how could I even think that? What do I do then?" Luckily, Lisa looked for help. Others do not. There are some things you can do, but they may not guarantee success. If your friend or family member is unable to begin alone you might want to stand beside her initially. Continue to be firm and offer to go with her to the first counseling session. Push her to get a complete physical exam and hopefully speak to a family doctor. Try to get her to go with you to an Overeaters Anonymous meeting where she will certainly find that she is not only not alone, but will likely hear her own story from someone else and will be made aware that there is hope. These meetings can also be a valuable resource for finding good professional help. Your offer to accompany her may be just the boost your friend needs.

Be Realistic

If your efforts are still met with refusal, don't give up, but maintain a more realistic estimate of what you alone can do. Consider breaking confidence and asking other supportive people for help. You are also not alone and may not need to be if efforts to seek help fail. You are probably a good friend and have been asked to maintain confidence, but this is a case where keeping a friend's secret can result in death. If you are a teenager, speak to a trusted adult as soon as possible. If possible, speak to your friend's parents. Perhaps you can speak to your own parent, a teacher, coach, school nurse or counselor, or priest, minister, or rabbi. They have likely handled similar situations in the past and may be able to advise you on what to do. They will also help you to decide, if it is a difficult situation, how to go to the friend's parents, and in some cases, may be willing to speak to the friend's parents themselves.

An ANRED website provides the following wonderful quote: "Life does not run like a TV show where some compassionate parent/friend/lover/pastor/counselor/doctor/says just the right thing so that the victim/sufferer sees the light and makes a 180° turn right before the last commercial. Life is complicated and messy. We don't have roadmaps and scripts to follow, but we do have multiple opportunities to choose wisdom and integrity over blind adherence to destructive patterns. Good luck on your journey!"

Lisa has indeed begun her journey to recovery, as she has come to the realization that self-help is not the answer. I hope that, at this point, Lisa's story has helped you to understand some of what may have felt frightening, confusing, and unpredictable. I hope that you have begun to realize that you are neither bad, unworthy, or really very different. Most important, you can reach out—you are not alone! There is help! In my next chapter, I will discuss just how to seek help.

8. Weekly Therapy
19 YEARS OLD

English Class Journal
5:05–5:20 P.M.
Shit! Perry is just like Dad. I picked a boy just like him. One who will never tell me he loves me. And that's what I really want to hear, isn't it? I can give a lot of bull about how it doesn't matter, he "shows" it when he looks at me, touches me, caresses me. But still, deep down, if he really does love me, why doesn't he tell me so? Once. I feel unlovable. But it's a conflict. I feel like I should be lovable, but I'm not. I'd still be surprised if he told me he loved me. Even though deep down that's what I tell myself is true and he briefly mentioned it a year ago. Who am I talking about now? Initially, Perry, but it could be either.

I don't know what this means or what, if anything, to do. But it's there, a piece to a puzzle, a puzzle I didn't even know existed.

English Class Journal
11:15–11:30 A.M.
Something hit me the other day, like a ton of bricks so to speak. It is silly, not to mention stupid, to do things now and have the future be your main motivator. What a waste. Now is all the time that is real. I don't want to throw it away.

Take Perry, for instance (anytime, anywhere). I came close to falling into foolhood. How do I know what the future will hold? For some reason, I was not thoroughly enjoying the time we have now in order to placate some future time. Ridiculous. Who knows? We may not end up with each other. For life. But we do have now, or whatever time we spend together.

When he said he very well might join ROTC, go into the Air Force or immigrate to Israel someday, not quite panic, but a scary feeling, an empty numbness came over me. It was hard enough, this being the first time we saw each other since my letter, without having to hear this kind of stuff. It's the first time the future didn't seem quite set. What if our lifestyles and dreams are completely, irrevocably, out of sync? We look at lots of things from different viewpoints. He's very righteous and idealistic.

So, I said, for once, don't think, worry, or plan about the future. Just relax and enjoy right now. Learn from and experience right now. It was a nice change of pace.

APRIL 15

English Class Journal
3:10–3:25 P.M.
I don't feel very good. What should I do? How should I do it? I don't feel guilty about the sexual feelings anymore. With Greg the other night, I've never been in that position before. He seems so blasé. Deep down I wanted to turn him on, and I did more than ever. But not enough. I've never been in the role of seductress or initiator before. Of course, he initiated it as always. But I'm the one who put my body close against his.

And, finally, he put his hand atop my shirt, but not enough! I wanted to lead him over to the couch and lie down. But didn't. Why did I feel this way? Maybe it's because he seems so mildly interested. It's not that I'm even thrilled to death while it's happening, although last time I did get turned on when he was pulling me closer.

I do find him sexy and extremely attractive. Perry and he are total opposites, sexually, at least. It was as if Greg wanted to be kissed, but I'm used to being the one who gets kissed and etc. Well, it's teaching me something.

APRIL 16

English Class Journal
9:20–9:35 A.M.
Why is it that nothing has ever counted unless I told my parents? It didn't matter that I talked to or went out with Perry unless they knew. I had to subtly let them know that Greg had been here on Saturday. I can't be getting better in bulimia counseling or my group therapy unless they know the progress. Grades don't matter unless they know. It's not just enough that I know. What's the big deal if I know? Sometimes I try to just keep it to myself. But I never do. I always end up telling them in one way or another.

It's as if I am trying to prove something to them. It dawned on me that I'm putting too much importance on what others think and not enough on how I feel, then I feel resentful over that and end up eating. I know what's right for me. I know if I'm in sync. I don't want to have to look to others or put others ahead of me when it comes to defining ME.

APRIL 17

I was inspired to write this when Greg fell asleep very late the other night in my apartment on the couch lying down with his head on my lap while the space shuttle was blasting off live on TV.

HEAD: Men Make the *Strangest* Bedfellows!

BYLINE: Lisa Messinger; Sophomore, Broadcast Journalism

I've done it on a water bed. I've done it on a twin bed. I've done it on a king-size. I've done it on a queensize. I've done it in a sleeping bag. I've even done it on a cot. Call me naïve. Call me out of it. Call me a virtual ignoramus. But I just don't see what the big deal is. It seems to me that one of the most overrated, overemphasized of our American pastimes has got to be going to bed with someone.

Maybe it's me. I know that after my friends have slept with someone they often feel as though they've had an exhilarating, sometimes thrilling, and, once in a while, spine-chilling experience. Not me.

Why is this? It's certainly not for lack of trying. My quest began when I was still a bright-eyed prepubescent. An idealistic romantic at heart, I decided to sleep only with someone who I loved and, more importantly, loved me: Greggy Pinsk. Greggy Pinsk was my first heartthrob not to mention bedfellow. We had been planning our rendezvous for weeks. It was at the joint Brownie/Cub Scout campout and nature awareness retreat. When our night finally arrived, we sneaked away from the campsite with sleeping bags in hand and dreams in heart.

I became quickly disenchanted, however. The most thrilling sensation I experienced was catching my finger in the zipper when we were zipping our sleeping bags together. After that, it was all downhill. I was awakened by the pine needles puncturing my derriere, the caterpillar crawling up my nose and the dew covering my entire body. It was then that I began to wonder what all the fuss was about.

One of my more recent ventures left me just as bewildered. Being a young college co-ed, I was living in my own off-campus apartment complete with termites and lumpy sofa bed. Buzz Giblet was my current flame. When I kissed Buzz and saw rockets, I felt a renewed sense of hope. However, when I realized that this was just the space shuttle blasting off on television I also realized that there was no real hope for me. I was right. Throughout the night Buzz snored, sneezed, burped, and made a number of less identifiable noises. He tossed and turned and, in the process, kicked me in the face with his work boot. I lost two teeth and any further desire to sleep with anyone ever again.

With this decision came another one: I'll be joining the convent next month. While I may be the first Jewish nun, it certainly seems to beat the alternative.

APRIL 17

English Class Journal
5:00–5:15 P.M.

I'm an "ex." I used to do it. I don't do it anymore. It's a part of the past. Since I am not doing it now, it's a part of my past. I never have to do it again. That activity and mode of self-expression is now over. Yes, over. Gone. No more. I have stopped. I am clean, straight. It's past tense. On April 16, peace was declared.

Not ignorant enough to believe that discontinuing the activity is the road to happiness. No more. This is a complex issue. To be dealt with. I realize now that this was a catchall for every problem. What do I really want? What do I really need?

There are things about myself that I didn't realize. That I was eating in response to. No more. At least the eating part. I'll have to look at the other part. And that takes guts.

APRIL 17

English Class Journal
5:15–5:30 P.M.

I have been disassociating. Put hair spray on my hair. Hair looked good. Put hair spray on again. Same result. Therefore, hair spray equals pretty hair. I lost touch with what my hair really looked like. All that mattered was that the hair spray was on. Then the hair must look good, right? Looking good, too. Make-up had to go on a certain way. Exactly. Then I look good, right?

If I put only certain quantities of food into my body and exercise it a number of times exactly, then that makes it look good, too. If I don't do this stuff, there is no way I can look good. I had really stopped looking at myself. It's easier to just do x and get y than have to deal with an unknown.

Last night I couldn't believe that I looked pretty, my face, even though I wasn't eating well. How can this be? It doesn't follow. Or does it?

Wake up! Be realistic. Your mind has been playing tricks on you. That was my way of life: Do this and this and this and you get this. Sometimes that may be true, but not all the time. So what are you going to do? Well, of course, realization is a crucial first step. I'm going to try and identify it in my life. I've got to learn to live with myself on a much less rigid basis.

APRIL 20

English Class Journal
10:40–10:55 A.M.

I don't want to be around people. I don't want people to look at me. Why? It's simple. I don't want to look at myself. I asked myself, if I never had to see any-

one, ever, would I still care how I looked? Maybe not. However, I would probably care how I felt, if I was sick or healthy. If you're fat, you feel differently,
unhealthy. So, I would care. When I lost that weight last summer, I used to be
able to say, to hell with what *they* think. I know I'm good, and that's all that
matters. I don't do that now because I don't have that same feeling of self-validation. If I did, I'd say to hell with them.

I like looking good. It gives me satisfaction. I don't feel I look good now. I
don't do it as much for others as I do it for my own sense of accomplishment
and progress. I do it to feel good about myself. I've learned that there's more to
me, though. More that has to be dealt with and felt good about. Okay. Fine. But
that doesn't mean I shouldn't care about how I look. It's important to me. I've
been letting it slide. A lot. One hundred twenty-eight pounds!! And I don't feel
good about that part of myself because of it.

I don't want to get fanatical. I don't want to punish myself. God, I'm not
punishing myself. I'm just taking Easy Street.

If I could lose weight as fast by eating, I would. I wouldn't not eat to punish myself. So there. One back-of-the-mind theory smashed.

I don't like being overweight. So, I will lose weight. Just because I've stopped
binging doesn't mean that I understood why I did it in the first place. First, it's
a cover-up. Second, it's a habit.

So, I'll try and figure out what it's covering up. Plus, use behavior modifi-
cation to break the habit part.

APRIL 20

English Class Journal
11:00–11:15 A.M.

Sex. What does it mean to me? This may also be one of the cover-ups. If I had
what I thought was a terrific body, I'd want to flash it around. Maybe. I guess I
don't want to have to deal with that. If I don't like my body, I don't have to see
anyone and, therefore, don't have to worry.

I never admitted I had sexual feelings and desires. That I like it. Who me?
Yes, under the right circumstances. Which are? Me. Looking and feeling terrific. That's what scares me: If I feel comfortable enough with me, I may not wait
around for Prince Charming (or Perry Schwartz, for that matter). I know it's normal to have sexual feelings, but it's easier not to make any decisions. I don't
feel sexual at all when I don't like how I look. But I know if I liked how I looked
then I would feel sexual. Of course, I wouldn't even kiss just anyone. However,
I know I'd be more curious than I am now. Like Greg, for instance, we know
each other so well. We're more than platonic. If I felt more confident, I'd like to
go further with him.

And I know I'd be more relaxed with Perry. I'd be able to be the one to start something instead of just lying there like a dead fish. Why am I scared of this? What can I do?

This little place. This little studio. At least it's mine, mine alone. Fifteen minutes from campus. Miles and miles from home. Fully furnished (yuk). It's mine. I still have that need to be alone. No roommate. No dorm mates. No family. God, for the week and a half I was at my parents' house after I gave Perry my letter, I felt like I was under guard. Eyes on me at all times. I told my mom, but that was it. I felt jumpy every minute, like they were thinking I was going to drop out of school again. All the money down the drain again. At least that's what I felt from my dad who barely spoke to me. Every night I just went right up to my room after I got home from school. Sitting down in the living room with them, I felt like I might jump out of my skin. I couldn't talk. I felt like I might cry or explode.

Well, here I am, just me. Me, just me, and my thoughts.

English Class Journal
10:45–11:00 P.M.

Tomorrow I start the seven-day quick weight-loss reducing program. Well, I start the preliminary two-day fruit juice cleansing fast.

I think I can fast for two days knowing that on the third day I can have some of that balanced good food I bought. Sixty dollars worth! It looks balanced and filling and interesting. And you can lose between ten and fifteen pounds in that reducing week.

I didn't want to go back to my old balanced eating. Even though I could have lost weight. I wanted an easy way to lose this fat, which is not me! That was too slow. I would stop eating nutritiously and then just end up gorging. It was not working.

This is a compromise. I can eat healthily and be full and still lose weight quickly.

As for keeping it off, I may like it enough to expand on it. Or if I go back to my 1,000–1,200 calorie plan that should maintain it.

Omitting, of course, binging. I have to deal with that. But I'm not going to be able to if I feel like I'm fat.

When I feel better about how I look, I think I'll be less driven and have a better perspective.

English Class Journal
6:15–6:30 P.M.

A nice-looking stranger just said hi to me. What is it that happens when I feel in control? Because I'm certainly not skinny, just as when I thought I was fat, I wasn't. What is it? I'm sitting here (college library) drinking strawberry nectar.

Dawned on me, I eat to cop out. If I didn't demand such rigidity from myself, then I wouldn't need to cop out. I could just plain live, experience, and enjoy.

How? Well, one way to start is to listen and follow my inner signals. About work. Trust myself. I'll do it. Twenty-four hours is enough time. I want to trust myself and give myself more leeway.

I'm a good kid. And, besides, sometimes I like to be "doing." I'm really not lazy. But I do need time to relax, rest, and be leisurely. I have to give this to myself.

Listen and Trust.

"INVENTORY"

Eight pieces of wheat bread with margarine (afternoon)

Supermarket trip: (late P.M.)
granola clusters (box)
granola bars (box)
diet ice cream (quart)
diet candy (box)

Burger King: (later P.M.)
1 Whopper with cheese
1 chicken sandwich
1 ham and cheese sandwich
2 small Cokes/1 small Dr. Pepper
large fries/onion rings

(Monday. A lot of Chinese Food.)

Philosophy 100, University of Southern California
Lisa Messinger

> If our actions are not completely under our
> control, are we morally responsible for them?

YAHTZEE!! I feel as though I have scored an emotional and unexpected Yahtzee. The dice that I threw, however, represent more than just the plastic playing pieces of a cardboard game. They signify facets of my life; and they have finally come together. It is as if I have been trapped in a mental Yahtzee game. I knew the straights, full houses, doubles, and triples. I was not, however, consciously aware of the importance, or even the existence, of a Yahtzee roll. With hindsight, though, I can look back and see that it was an unconscious desire for that very Yahtzee that motivated many of my actions.

I am referring analogously to my 11-year bout with bulimia, the binging-purging eating disorder. I thought I knew why I chose this behavior. I thought it was a conscious choice, one of my own free will. Recently, however, with the help of a therapist, I realized this was not the case. My motivator has actually been feelings and desires that I had repressed. The fact that I had felt unloved by my father was something I never, ever admitted to myself on a conscious level. Yet, now it seems clear that that has been what prompted some of my bulimic actions. I was surprised and confused. If my actions were not completely under my control, not completely free according to philosophical definition, was I still responsible, morally or otherwise, for what I had done to myself? After careful deliberation, I feel the answer is yes. I examined both my unconscious motivations, which I did not have control over, and the conscious actions that they led to, which I did have control over. I conclude that any tangible results, those for which I would be responsible or not responsible, occurred directly because of my conscious actions regardless of what my subliminal motivations may have been. Although this is only one case, the logic used can be applied to other instances where responsibility is questionable.

So far, I have stated that unconsciously I was unfree. It is necessary to examine this more carefully, however. For, if I were both consciously and unconsciously free then there would be no question as to my responsibility. However, my unconscious behavior does not coincide with definitions of freedom. If we use Harry G. Frankfurt's conclusive definition in "Freedom of the Will and the Concept of a Person" as a base, my conduct appears to be unfree. Frankfurt contends that an act, A, is free if and only if it was caused by a desire to do A such that one, the agent wanted to act upon the desire to do A more than any other desire he had at the time; and two, his priorities were shaped by reason and awareness and with a sensibility to the consequences. Let A equal my action, which was eating. The agent, me, did *not* want to act upon the desire to do A more than any other desire I had at the time. On the contrary. Action A was merely a substitute for my real desire, to feel loved. I convinced myself that my top priority was to eat when it was not. As a result, my priorities were not shaped by reason and awareness and certainly not with a regard for the consequences. Since I was not fulfilling my top priority, a need for love, the consequence would inevitably be more eating in an attempt to fulfill this desire. But since I was unaware of this desire in the first place, I could have no idea as to the consequences. My priorities, therefore, were shaped by deception and fear and were consequently unfree.

However, it is precisely because of this deception that I can say that I am responsible for all of the results of this destructive eating pattern. Because of this unconscious delusion, my conscious action, eating, can be seen as a free action. When I actually ate, I was in accordance with Frankfurt's definition of freedom. On a conscious level, I had one desire that topped all others: the desire to put food into my body. This was not only a strong desire, it was a priority. I also had other desires. I wanted to lose weight, but I wanted to eat more. I wanted to do homework, but I wanted to eat more. I even wanted not to binge, but I wanted to binge more. I was also aware of what I was doing. I was breaking my personal code. I was doing something wrong, I knew this. I was also very good at employing reason: I need this for energy; I didn't eat yesterday, so there's no harm in gorging today; peanut butter is not a solid food. I also had the consequences in mind: I would gain weight; I would be disgusted with myself; I would probably do it again or starve as a result. Consciously, therefore, according to Frankfurt, I was free.

A single action, therefore, can be unfree in some respects and free in other respects. The question we are concerned with here is which respect deals with the aftereffects, the tangible results. Needless to say, if it were the unfree aspect that led to the results, the agent should not be held responsible. On the other hand, if it were the free aspect that led to these results, then the agent could be held responsible. In my case, there is a disguised action and a clear action. The disguised action is an unconscious attempt to block out feelings of being unloved by filling or masking the gap with food. The clear action is the conscious eating for superficial reasons. The results of the disguised action are inconclusive. I do not get love; but this is not negative since I didn't know I wanted it. The results of the action, eating, however, are recognizable, weight gain and disgust. These are the results of bulimia for which I would either be responsible or not responsible. These are results of the free aspect of the action. Therefore, I am responsible for these results.

Although this may seem isolated, it can be applied to other cases. People often delude themselves. Therefore, unconsciously, because they do not know their true desires, they are unfree. Consciously, however, they do know what they are doing, although it may be for misguided reasons, as a result of their delusion. They are consequently free in this respect. Even though they are under a delusion, they are aware of the impending results. Therefore, although they are not totally free, they are, nevertheless, responsible for these consequences. (Grade received: A)

APRIL 23

English Class Journal
6:20–6:35 P.M.
I don't think of other people as seeing me as a person. Now I understand better why I avoid people and eat instead of dealing with them. I feel like they

only see me by how I look and what I do, not what I am. Maybe it's because I've judged myself that way a lot. If I do good and look good, I don't have to look inside. Is it related to Dad? Do I feel that he doesn't know or wouldn't like me as a person? He just knows my accomplishments and the outer crust, how I look. He doesn't know the rest. How do I change this view I have? What do I do?

I asked myself, if I were alone on a desert island, would I care about how I looked? First I thought, well, there's no reason for it, but, then I realized that I would care about how I physically felt. The shape you're in and the food you eat have to do with this, but it's not how you look. So my desire now is more to feel good.

Most of the time when I eat it's to "cop out" of something. Maybe I put too much pressure on myself, do expect perfection, and if I would relax and listen, really listen, to myself, I wouldn't want or feel a need to cop out.

There is no future for Perry and me. We don't want the same kind of lives. And I don't want him (if I could have him). I never think it, but I don't like our relationship now. I clung to the idea of "someday." There is no someday. There is no now. It's over.

APRIL 23

English Class Journal
11:00–11:15 P.M.

Could it be that all the dieting, rigidity of exercise, etc., is a cover-up? Since I binge, I have to do all of those other things to be okay. In my mind, that's the only way I could ever be okay, right? Why, why is it just me? There must be people who are thin who just eat and moderately exercise whenever they want. It seems so incomprehensible to me to picture a life where I would just live and not follow a definite plan. I never questioned my structure before.

Maybe it would just happen if I let it. Maybe it's what I thought, because I expect such rigid adherence to these plans, I can't do it, so I have to "cop out." IRONY. I make the plan in the first place to stop, refrain from, and forbid the eating and then it's this very plan that causes me to turn to eating. I'm crying now. I think I've really hit something.

This is scary because it pulls the whole rug out from my way of life. I never questioned my methods. I never knew why I couldn't follow them.

Maybe I don't need a plan like that. The time I stopped binging it seemed like things just started happening. I felt like I was losing weight without "willing" it to happen. Lately, I've realized I've made my life a prison sentence. Do this now. Do this next. Do this. Do this. What should I do? Now I feel lost.

I was making myself diet. I was making myself exercise. It was not directly because I wanted to feel good, or felt like it, or for any really rational reasons. I was (am) doing it because I *had to*. Why is that? I want to eat and exercise when I want to and for a reason. In the back of my mind, I knew what I was doing didn't make any sense. I was putting so much true energy into the diet and exercise for what I thought were obvious reasons, to lose weight and look good, and yet I was putting just as much energy into frenzied eating. I knew the two were canceling each other out. And didn't fit. Somehow I feel that if I stop the binging I won't need that superhuman effort in order to feel good or look okay. Eventually I just would. That spells relief with a capital "R." But is it true?

APRIL 24

Well, the lid has finally blown off. The cover is blown. It's all out in the open now. All the blood and guts are on the floor.

Well, Dad already knew. I mean we had to tell him in order to afford psychotherapy from Francine every week. I didn't go into much detail. It was hard enough to tell something to someone you know won't understand in order to get money. And, by all appearances, he didn't understand. He'd never heard of it.

"I sometimes eat 5 or 10 cookies after dinner, even if I'm on a diet, and I feel bad," he said. "But I stop. Why don't you just stop yourself? So, you've got a sweet tooth."

Sweet tooth. I'll show you sweet tooth. When they came over today, after my crying conversation on the phone for the first time with my mom that my dad did not love me, I knew I was finally ready to say something. I couldn't stand it anymore. I realized a big part of my problem, it was trapped in me, and it had to come out.

So when my dad antagonized me by saying again how when he saw ice cream cartons or cookie boxes under my bed at home he thought I just had a sweet tooth and that I didn't want anyone to know about it, and besides, I was always so touchy and preoccupied with my looks, and always going up to my room when I was living at home growing up, he just didn't want to upset me by bringing it up.

"Upset me!" I said crying. "You want to see what a sweet tooth I have?" I hadn't thrown out the trash of yesterday's binge. I happened to have it hidden in the closet in a shopping bag: a medium pizza box, a bag of potato chips, a pint of ice cream, candy wrappers, junk food cartons. "This is not just a sweet tooth," I kept yelling.

"Okay, okay," he said. "I can see that."

I'm sorry I made my mom hysterical. Although I wasn't too far from hysteria myself. "We'd love you no matter what, no matter what," she kept crying.

When I said I thought he wouldn't love me no matter what, he said, "You and your brother are the most important things in the world to me." *Things?*

"But you wouldn't love me, I feel, unless I look perfect and do perfect in school," I said.

"That's ridiculous," he said.

"You wouldn't love me no matter what," I said.

Ah. The zinger. The million dollar question.

"How can I write you a blank check for my love?"

"Oh, my God." (Mom)

"What do you mean?" (Me)

"What if a kid robbed a bank or was a mass murderer and went to the electric chair? How do you love them then?" he said.

"Oh, my God, I'd love my child no matter what they did." (Mom)

"I'm not talking about *anyone,* I'm talking about me," I said. "You've known me for 19 years, you can't bet yet that I won't be a killer or a criminal? I'm talking about *me.*"

"Still, how can anyone write a blank check with love?"

"Don't you see you're telling me there's a line I can't cross over? I don't know where it is. I believe that line to be not getting straight A's or looking perfect."

"That's ridiculous."

"Why? You say you wouldn't love me no matter what. How am I supposed to know where the line is drawn?"

"How can you say that to her?" (Mom)

"So, you can't tell me that there's nothing *I* could do in my life, the life you already know, that wouldn't make you stop loving me?"

Incredulously from Mom, "You can't tell her you know her well enough to know you'll always love her?"

"I guess so."

We brought dinner in and ate. He said, "You won't need this [shopping bag] anymore, will you?" And threw it out.

So, what can I say? In a way, I'm relieved. I am not crazy. I was *right.* I had a parent who did feel the way I thought he did. I thought, how could my feelings be right? And yet, now I see, to some degree, I was right. That gives, I suppose, some validity to the disgusting actions that have been masking all these years the way I really felt. Of course, this can't be the sole explanation. There must be other reasons, too. But, nevertheless, I feel as though a brick is off my head.

I've upset my whole family. The family I've tried so hard not to upset before. I wasn't crazy.

English Class Journal
6:00–6:15 P.M.

About Perry. It is so confusing to me that I could have been doing things—seemingly important things—without ever truly questioning my motives, or if it's the best thing to do.

Without really admitting it, I thought I wanted this relationship for the "future." We were waiting for something to happen. That's why I had to "settle" for now, and eat and eat and eat to push down my real feelings. However, I never even thought honestly or deeply about whether or not I even wanted a future with him. I just assumed, "He's certainly good enough. He's probably *it.*"

But he's not what I want. I do like him right now, at this point in time, but not for the long run. We don't want the same things out of life. He also seems so condescending without even trying to be. Like he'll put up with my "kooky" eating behavior. Well, gee, thanks. I don't want to be put up with. I want to be loved, accepted, and understood.

And I don't really like his snobbishness around other people, his righteousness, or his highly moral attitude. He's narrow-minded. I think that's sad.

I want more than he is. There is no future. There is no now. Perry and Lisa are coming to an end.

SUICIDE WAS THE WRONG CHOICE

BY LISA MESSINGER

Sarah was a friend of mine. Not a close friend. But close enough for me to know that her recent suicide was a mistake. Some might say that suicide is always a mistake. Maybe. This one was.

Sarah thought she knew everything. She didn't. She was sure there was nothing "out there" for her. She was wrong. She was a high school senior. She didn't know there was life after high school graduation or, for that matter, after college graduation or marriage or med school or thirty.

Sarah, if you can hear me, there's something I'd like to say. If you can't, maybe someone else will. If no one should hear, I will. I'll learn to appreciate my own problematic existence, because life can always change.

Sarah, you did it at the wrong time. It was such a waste, because you didn't know. You just didn't know. Life isn't high school, Sarah. Far from it. Of course, while we're there, it's hard to realize that there's more. That it's better. That it's different. But it is. If only you would have let yourself find out.

Why couldn't you have waited? Why did you think that you had all the answers? Answers that you felt couldn't or wouldn't solve your problems. Why couldn't you have waited and found out that sometimes problems just seem to pass away with time? And when they don't, nothing is insurmountable, Sarah. Nothing!

I know you think that I think your problems didn't go beyond broken prom dates, perennial second places, and unfinished term papers. You're wrong. I know. Oh, I don't know exactly. But I do know that your disturbances went much deeper.

But, Sarah, what leaves me so incredibly angry and empty is that had you waited, you would have probably discovered something, growing up brings with it strength. Your problems may not have gone away, but you would have fought them or, at least, accepted them. I know you would have.

Just as I know that you, Sarah, the perennial people pleaser would have eventually become your own person. One day you would have woken up and known that your own opinion was more important than that of your parents, than that of your friends, than that of anyone. You would have realized that you alone control your life. And, Sarah, at that moment you would have grabbed control. You would have come alive.

Sarah, why the hell did you have to be so intelligent and mature? I see it in so many mature and intelligent people; you think you know it all. You may know a lot, but *nobody* knows it all. Your world may have been falling apart yesterday. It may be rotten today. But as for tomorrow, next week, or next month, who's to say?

Sarah, I have to say it, you were so damned ignorant. I know. I felt miserable through most of high school, too. Now I can see that my vision was terribly limited, almost blinded. I would never have guessed that only months later, I would have a dream job, totally new friends in college and at that job, and, most importantly, a completely revised and more realistic image of myself.

I have come full circle, Sarah. Unfortunately, you circumvented yourself. I didn't know what was in store for me. It just happened. You thought you knew what was in store for you. It's too bad that you were wrong. Too bad and too late.

Lisa Messinger is a sophomore majoring in broadcast journalism.

[This was published at this time in the *Daily Trojan,* the University of Southern California student newspaper and, then, after graduation, syndicated to other regular newspapers.]

MAY 1

I have been exaggerating my life. I have been grouping my whole life into one category, weight.

It seems so ridiculous now.

Unreal.

MAY 2

MY LIFE HAS BEEN ONE BIG TRADE OFF. I HAVE BEEN EATING INSTEAD OF LIVING!

I see now that my belief that other people didn't have trust in me was paranoid. It was a sign trying to tell me or show me that I wasn't trusting my own self.

MAY 4

I'm going to be okay,
not because I'm going to *make* myself be okay,
but because I'm going to *let* myself be okay.

9. Skipping Sessions

19 YEARS OLD

DAILY TROJAN

I WAS A TEENAGE FRESCA FREAK

BY LISA MESSINGER

"Buuurrp!" The dead silence was broken by an incredibly picturesque belch. Every eye turned from its midterm to the culprit—me. I could hide neither the embarrassment on my face, nor the Diet Pepsi on my breath—the secret was out. I felt like the words "Nutrasweet junkie" were written all over me.

It all started innocently enough. I had needed to pull an all-nighter, however, my eyes weren't cooperating. Unwittingly, I swallowed my Vivarin tablet with a Diet Rite chaser. The pill wore off; the dietetic daze didn't. The next morning, I found myself craving Diet Coke and Wheaties for breakfast.

My life became a relentless journey from soda machine to soda machine. I cashed in all of my paper money in order to support my habit. In a Nutrasweet-stupor, I sailed from the SAS basement to the college library lobby to the Student Union, where they have two. This eliminates the convulsions and epileptic-type attacks that can occur when there's only one machine and the dreaded "Out of Order" sign appears.

However, diet soda is only the beginning. It can lead to even more severe abuse. I needed the hard stuff. I began popping dietetic jellybeans between classes. Washing them down with Diet 7-Up was my biggest mistake. I woke up in a hospital emergency room having my stomach pumped.

By this time, however, my addiction was so strong I couldn't stop. I had to get "sweet" all the time, and the jellybeans weren't working anymore. Snorting dietetic gelatin became my favorite, not to mention only, pastime. People started questioning my inflamed nostrils. Actually, this was only the residue from raspberry, my favorite flavor.

I realized I had a problem. However, I thought I was the only one. Oprah Winfrey saved my life. I saw her interviewing a reformed diet-food junkie. My habit could be kicked! That day, I made the most important phone call of my life. "Hello, Sugar Substituters Anonymous, my name is Lisa M., and I'm an artificial sweetener abuser." Since then, I've been abstinent. However, I still carry a few packets in my purse—just in case.

Lisa Messinger is a sophomore majoring in broadcast journalism.

MAY 8	
Weight: 129$^1/_2$	Desired Weight: 120
Week One, May 8: 129$^1/_2$	Week Three, May 22:
Week Two, May 15:	Week Four, May 29:

Breakfast:
1 egg
1 slice wheat bread
1/2 grapefruit

Snack:
1 apple

Lunch:
3 oz. hamburger
1 1/2 oz. white cheese

Italian sauce
1 slice French bread
dinner salad (Thousand Island dressing
on the side)

Double Treat:
1 family-size candy bar
1 family-size raspberry-filled candy bar
1 single-serving banana cream pie
A little chocolate ice cream and a mini
chocolate cream pie

STOP THIS, YOU STUPID FOOL!!!

MAY 8

2:15 A.M.

I am looking in the mirror. Blob! Not fat. But not nice either. Rounded, expanded stomach. Jellylike, hanging boobs. Face that's quickly losing shape. Strangely shaped butt, like the muscles are in the wrong place. Thighs with a larger circumference. Same with upper arms. Hips curved. Waist wide. Not fat and not ugly, but certainly icky! I *feel* it all the time, this extra weight. Probably about 130 now. I want to feel healthy, vital, and in tune with my body.

It's not affecting much but my body image, though. I still feel strong and good about other things.

But how we *feel* and how we look is something we have to deal with all the time. It's what we are.

Now, thank goodness, nothing else is wrapped up with my body and weight. So, it can go away without confusing me and setting me up.

Bye, bye.

MAY 8

3:00 A.M.

I don't like the way my body looks. I was going to say I don't like the way I look, but that's not altogether true. I look heavier, but not ugly or homely. I have a nice face. I like the way it looks better when it's thinner, though.

I see now that eating nutritionally is not the only route. I could be (and was being these last six weeks) a haphazard, imbalanced eater. Whether or not I gained weight, I didn't feel guilty. However, I also didn't feel good! I got headaches, stomachaches, and even threw up. That was after I had a bacon quiche followed by almost a pint of double chocolate chip ice cream. It seems these last weeks I've been trying to prove to myself that it's okay to eat anything

I want. I'm talking *anything.* Candy everyday. Big family-size bars. Fast food everyday. Everything I forbade myself before, and then ended up binging on. Now I'm just eating it everyday, whenever I want, without guilt, and without the purging of starvation the next days or excessive forced exercise. And, I've been gaining weight.

Now I'm beginning to see there is a reason to eat nutritiously, and it isn't to lose weight or torture yourself. It's to be healthy and feel healthy.

God, I've been through an emotional and physical wringer. It's very recent that I've thought thinness is only physical and doesn't really mean anything else.

I do have confidence in my intelligence. In myself. My basic attractiveness. My sense of humor. My writing. I'm a good friend. A nice, caring, empathetic person. Good worker, sensitive, ambitious, loving, lovable, sweet, special, wonderful, beautiful, normal person.

I know this *now,* and this doesn't change with physical changes.

MAY 10

Well, I don't want to be fat anymore. One-hundred-and-thirty-one pounds! I'm going and that's all there is to it. I can't wait anymore. I have to do something now.

School. Well, I'll miss a mid-term tomorrow and, what am I saying, I'll miss the rest of the semester. I can't think straight. I'm going.

Three weeks at this reducing spa in the country. It's a lot of money, but I have it saved and want to use it. Maybe I can get back to normal.

I just can't live with this kind of fat on me.

MAY 11

Dear Lisa,

Whatever you choose to do in life, you will do well. I'm behind you all the way. I'm here whenever you need me.

I love you,
Mom

Dear Lisa,

You can take whatever suitcase you prefer. Hope you have a satisfying and enjoyable time at the reducing spa. We'll look forward to your call and seeing you when you get home. Hope you can make it for the concert we have tickets for at the Greek Theatre on the 30th. Maybe we can have a picnic dinner before the show.

Love,

Mom and Dad (signed in Dad's handwriting)

MAY 23

I rebelled. I stopped exercising. I started eating whatever I wanted. Even though I wasn't doing any of my "classical" binging, I was eating a lot. I didn't like the way I looked and didn't want to wait until school got out or I could get off work. I felt desperate and I ran. I ran to the health spa resort praying to melt back into my old, tolerable body.

I'm still associating other things with being thin, strength and an ability to deal with people strongly. I see that happening when I picture myself thin. And now, I'm not thin. I crawled back here after two days of a proposed three-week stay to go back to school (but not to work right away) and hide in my dim studio apartment, phone unplugged, door locked. I haven't gone out, to a movie, to a restaurant, to a party since—I can't even remember when—because I feel fat and isolated and confused and locked in my own dungeon of a mind.

I felt that by running away, doing something so drastic and out of line, by leaving everything and everyone in midstream, it would be like slapping people in the face and saying, "I'm not what you thought," and then when I got back, I could tell the truth.

MAY 24

English Journal
5:45–6:00 P.M.

My university group therapy for eating disorders ended today. It was exciting to be in the first one ever at USC. I felt it. Tears were in my eyes, but I also felt it inside. It wasn't as if I had been incredibly close to any one of them—Anita (the head of university's counseling services, who was our therapist), Jane, Melissa, Jill, Heather, or Kari—but, as Anita mentioned at the beginning, there was a closeness and a relationship within the group as a whole. I'm going to miss it, but I do feel that I won't close out the people in my life anymore. That group existed at a crucial time for me.

"Here Comes the Sun," that classic song is ringing in my ears. This is it, honey! You're coming out of a shell, a shell that was an incredibly cockeyed mind. So much has changed. You've discovered so much. Had so many insights. Learned a lot. There have been ups and downs. It can't be all up. Some wonderful things have happened. You've met some interesting, special people. One of them being yourself. It was a mishmash. Things hidden deep under the surface. I don't know where I am or where I'm going, and it actually feels okay.

10. Promises, Promises

19 YEARS OLD

7:43 P.M.

As of June, I never binged again. My last binge on May 30 consisted of a medium sausage pizza and an order of spaghetti al pesto. My stomach hurt and my head throbbed and then it dawned on me, once again, that I never had to binge again. I could control this. There is a difference now, though. Stopping binging is just that. Nothing more. This is, of course, the key.

Now if I can only find the door, let alone the lock.

2:00 A.M.

WEIGHT: 140!!!!

I just started a fast. Obviously, that's the only way I'll get some results. No food will pass these lips. I am mad. I hate the state my life is in. Give it a week. Forget food. I'm not eating. Water, that's it. I want to drop at least ten pounds. Then, I'll see what to do. Fasting's okay. Other people do it. I really am absolutely disgusted, and it's time to *do* something. Really, *do* something. Nothing can make me eat.

I'll weigh myself for the first time in two days.

I blew it! I can't fast. Therefore, I will go on the diet Dad promotes and *only* eat these foods in order to make this disgusting weight go away.

- grapefruit
- protein bread
- low-fat cottage cheese
- carrots
- celery
- canned chicken
- cucumbers
- broccoli, string beans, green pepper
- turkey

(With him walking around the house talking about it all the time—now that I moved home again for the summer—I can at least try it. Maybe it'll help.)

JULY 1

Keep this fourteen-day chart of your weight loss while on the diet:
Week 1:

Day 1	Day 2	Day 3	Day 4	Day 5	Day 6	Day 7
131	128	128	$130\frac{1}{2}$	$129\frac{1}{2}$	$128\frac{1}{2}$	

Week 2:

Day 8	Day 9	Day 10	Day 11	Day 12	Day 13	Day 14

Took off _____ Pounds

JULY 13

Dear Lisa,

I know this letter is long overdue, but the most important letters I seem to put off because it takes too long to write down all my feelings. The not-so-personal letters are easier to write. Accept my apologies and get prepared for a long letter. Relax, have a soda, and sit back!

I came home all ready to tell my family about my bulimia, but chickened out. It seemed that there was never a time when everyone was together, and I lost my courage. I guess I still feel like I can lick this alone and don't need to burden them with more problems.

Actually, I'm hardly binging and vomiting at all, maybe once a week. From four times a day, that's quite a drop. I'm eating normal food, so maybe I don't need to binge and eat forbidden foods. I do throw up some of my meals if I feel I've eaten a tremendous amount. Overall, I'm doing better, and I'm feeling much better about myself. Things here have not gone well, but I'm reacting and showing my feelings and weaknesses instead of pigging out. Knowing that I can handle stressful situations and not fall apart has made me like myself so much more. Sure, there are times when I get so lonely or unhappy that I cry myself to sleep, but at least I'm not eating my blues away. I still have a long way to go, but maybe back at school with the group and a counselor I'll beat this totally.

I've been shopping a lot because it keeps me busy and out of the house. For once, I've actually been buying clothes instead of saying I'll wait until I lose weight.

Enough of me, how are you? Did you enjoy the spa? I would love to do that. How are you doing with your parents, especially your dad? Did you find an apartment or get housing from school? I haven't heard from Heather, have you? I really miss talking to you, Heather, and the rest of the group. Nowhere else can I admit all my problems and still be understood.

For instance, I can't talk to anyone here about Jack. We broke up when I got home. I was furious at myself for not telling him to get lost because no one has the right to treat me the way that he has. Also, my stepmother and father are having problems again. My brothers were all very upset, and I tried to help them without taking all the guilt on myself. Things are better, but I still think it's a little tense. I'd like to go in for family counseling, but no one else seems to like the idea. So, I'm keeping a diary and trying to verbalize my feelings instead of clamming up.

Anyway, I'll be back in L.A. August 12, and, during a break from moving in, I'll call you. Hopefully, we can get together before school starts. I can fix us lunch or dinner after I get settled, or maybe we can get together over a diet soda! Thanks for the support!

Love,
Jane

JULY 22

Dear Jane,

I'm sitting here backstage on a TV show answering their phones. Fun, but not all that exciting. The perfect time to write a letter! So you'll understand if this letter seems a little disjointed (from people and/or phone interruptions).

Your letter was a relief. Really. I felt like I was reading something that I could have written. Finally, I thought, someone who understands, and who I understand! I so miss you and the other members of the support group, but especially you! Over the summer, I've been feeling like you have. Lonely. Unhappy. A little confused and angry. And everything's going pretty okay, too.

Well, eatingwise, that is. Since I came back from the spa in Palm Springs (two months ago), I have not done any of my "classic" binges. I've pretty much eaten what I want. But, I got into the habit (ritual?) of eating whatever I wanted in the morning (pizza or whatever was in the house—but not binge-size portions, just single servings), and then I wouldn't eat during the day. I exercised, too, so I lost twelve of the twenty pounds I had gained. Since I wasn't depriving myself, I thought I had normalized my eating. But I'm really not sure. One good thing is that I haven't been feeling guilty over these foods, but I haven't eaten them in front of anyone else either.

A couple of weeks ago this didn't seem nutritious enough, though. So, I went on the diet my dad was on, but I was always hungry and didn't like it. For once, I went off a diet without guilt. I've decided if I want to eat a big meal in the morning (usually meat and bread), then it will be more balanced eating fruit and vegetables during the day.

The amazing thing is that every time I "willed" myself to stop binging in the past, it didn't work. Now, it's just gone. And, as I'm writing, I realize why. I'm not being a perfectionist. For once! I'm just letting myself do what I want.

I'm not "willing" weight loss either, and it's hard to do that when I'm not the weight I want to be. But, if I did "will" it, I know I'd gain instead of lose.

One thing I've realized, and it's been tough, is the value of real friends. I was lonely because I cut myself off from everyone for so long, and they didn't know why. Two good friends went back to the Midwest after school got out with me still not seeing them. I wrote them letters but was evasive. I didn't hear anything for a while, and I was depressed and mad at myself for being so destructive. Then, the day your letter came, Bob called from Wisconsin, where he's home for the summer. I felt semi-uplifted. I feel, though, that I've made my relationships with everyone somewhat strained.

When I went back to work after my spa-induced absence, no one had known where I was, or why, for those six weeks. I now feel funny with some people who had been friends. Even though I didn't stay at the spa and had returned home to go to school, I still was given the hiatus from work.

Also, friends from high school that I had "cut out" are drifting back. Two girls, especially, and I feel so foolish for letting our friendships slide. Right now I feel like I'm rebuilding everything.

When you wrote about you and Jack, I felt like you were talking about me and Perry. Although I haven't admitted it, I feel very hurt. Since I told him "about myself," I saw him once in April! There have been extenuating circumstances and, when we saw each other, we were as intimate physically as we always had been before, but I feel like he doesn't even care. I mean I told him in the letter I wrote him that I was sick and in pain and that I loved him, and from him I get nothing. Maybe it's just pride, because I felt only months ago that I was going to break it off with him. I feel like he's done it, and I wanted to be the one!

Which brings me to my next rejection story, Greg. We're both pages at the TV studio. We dated from July to April. I did nothing. He called and called and called. We talked a lot. We work together. I really liked him, although, at some points I thought our relationship was ridiculous. It was mainly platonic. I thought he kissed me because we started out that way. At one point, I told him this. He said, no, that wasn't the way it was, and so we continued. I never understood our relationship. I wrote him a letter from Palm Springs reminding him how much I liked him and hinting when I'd be home. After nine months of calling, he didn't. When I went back to work, I felt strange. Our first day together, like we have so many times, we got something to eat after work. When it was time to say good-bye, he didn't kiss me. I felt awful and dejected. Not so much for this one incident, but what it implied. It was a blatant non-gesture. We haven't said anything, but I feel like I've been semi-dumped by two desirable guys I had for two years and nine months, respectively. And no one even really dumped me.

Of course, I assumed both of them acted the way they did because of the way I looked. (Greg's standing here right now. In fact, he sat here for ten minutes asking me to whom I was writing. I had an urge to kick him. I don't get him. He probably doesn't get me either. Talk about up-to-the minute letters.)

Anyway, another gray area involves my dad. On the surface everything's "peachy," but I find myself feeling very mad and frustrated about him. When I came back from Palm Springs, he blew up at me for no real reason. (A floor cleaning man rang our doorbell and I slept through it. My brother did, too, but that, for some reason, was different.) He said he didn't like my attitude, or the type of person I'm becoming. He wanted to change me, he said. Even though I had confessed my longtime problem to him months ago, he asked me how I thought *he* felt when he saw me ten to fifteen pounds heavier. So he was going to get skinny just to show me. Because of my "attitude"—which I felt was honesty for once, and felt good about—he said I couldn't use the charge card or go to the bulimia psychologist I've been seeing since February. This whole thing seemed unbelievable to me. Jane, I didn't even do anything. It shows how insensitive he was to my misery by cutting off my therapy, my one outlet. The ironic thing is that the reason I slept through the doorbell is that I stayed up until 3:00 A.M. to jog around my pool, so that I could weigh less in the morning. I've been doing this every night, as I often did when I was in high school, and I've been tired every day, but, of course, I didn't tell my dad this.

(This guy just asked me to go water skiing on Saturday. He said he's been wanting to ask me out for a long time, but didn't. I gave him my number.) Anyway, I'm getting barraged with phone calls here at work. I wish I could write more because I want to ask all about you. So, write and tell me. I can't wait to see you, although I can wait to go back to school. (I'm going to have to commute from home instead of live at the dorm. I feel like I want to show my parents I'm "OK" before asking them to help me rent another apartment, even though they said I could.) Having you there will make it much, much more bearable. Take care.

Love,
Lisa

JULY 24

Lisa,

Well, it's about time I wrote this letter. How have you been? How is your work? I'm looking forward to coming back out to California in a few weeks and seeing you. I hope we can get together before school starts. My dad and I are driving out to L.A. We should arrive on the 24th and move into my apartment that afternoon. I'll call you at home that evening. If I can't get hold of you, you know where I'll be.

Unfortunately, I pulled a muscle in my calf while I was playing basketball. I'm going to be on crutches for a week, but I love all the attention I've been getting. My tennis game has improved since I got out of school. It shows that even though I'm a teaching pro, I should practice more myself! I hope I can go to two tournaments the last two weekends of the summer. I'll let you know how they turn out. I did win the singles league, and my friend and I came in second in mixed doubles. You and I should play some tennis before classes start.

I've been working about thirty hours a week this summer for that same engineering firm I worked for last summer. I'm ready to go back to school, though. After one year of difficult engineering studies, working in an office seems easy.

I can't wait to see you. I miss you.

Love,
Bob

P.S. I hope you are coping with your problem. I'm also glad you told me about it without, though, ever telling me what it is! I'm glad to hear it's not that serious, because I love you, and your friendship means a lot to me!

JULY 30

Dear Lisa,

I'm so glad my letter came at a good time for you. Yours came at a needy time, too. You feel I know and understand you, and I feel the same way about you! Sometimes, I can't believe how much alike we think.

I was happy to read how well you're doing with eating and losing weight. You're finally at a point where you can diet normally. I haven't gotten that far. I tried to go on a diet a few weeks ago, and, within a day, I was binging on "forbidden" foods. So, I stopped my diet plans and am doing better. I'm still eating a lot, but the guilt is fading. I really hate feeling this fat (I always do when I get up to 150 pounds), but I know if I try to starve or diet, I'll only end up vomiting again. My first reaction to your twelve-pound weight loss was jealousy and the feeling that I should lose weight. But then I realized that I don't have to compete with anyone. I also realized how much you have had to learn before you could "diet." So now I'm truly happy for you and know that one day I'll reach that point, too.

Your love life sounds exciting. You are too sensitive about your looks, especially if you keep getting asked out. You are beautiful outside and inside. Just keep remembering that. My love life, however, is not so smooth. Jack and I have not spoken at all since I wrote him from school. I know he won't call unless I do first, and I really don't want to call him. I'm happy without being around him all the time and realized how much I depended upon him for my self-esteem.

Lisa, about your dad, let me speak as the grad psych student I am. I think he's having a hard time adjusting to the new you. Before, you were the ideal daughter and weren't a threat. Now that he senses that you are changing, it may frighten him. I'm so relieved that you'll still be at school, even if you are going to live at home. You can come over to my apartment anytime between classes or to study or visit. Maybe we can arrange a time to go to the library together so you won't feel like you have nowhere to go.

About the family problems I mentioned in my last letter, I decided in the midst of all this that I could either take all the problems upon myself and go bananas, or I could love, support, and be concerned but not let it get to me. I chose to not let the problems get to me. I will never be able to solve the problems we have, and it's time I started to look out for my welfare and stop living for everyone else. In a sense, it's like being conceited. It really is more like self-respect and self-love. So I'm happy in spite of all that's been going on, something that's unusual for me.

Well, Lisa, it's almost my bedtime. Only one more day of getting up early for my part-time summer job. I can't wait to see you. Keep up the spirits. You're such an inspiration to me.

Love,
Jane

AUGUST 8

I have been reconfirmed. My faith in life has been renewed. I feel alive again. Much more so than before. Wherever this goes, I have gotten something important from it.

I've learned to trust my feelings. All the time I tried to deny them about this person and push them away, they were still there. I see that I can still have strong, potent feelings after these months of bulimia drought.

Right now, emotion and confusion fill my mind: I feel like I may be falling in love. The last time I felt that way with Perry it was true. This time, though, I'm a lot more confused. I'm just not sure. I've been pushing the feelings down for so long about this particular fellow TV page, they're all mushed up.

Brent is . . . dynamic, sweet, sensitive, cute, handsome, intelligent, talented, funny, witty, going everywhere at once. I admire him, like him a lot, and may even . . .

He thinks I'm wonderful! Special, pretty, sweet. I really do feel terrific when I'm around him. It's not that he "makes" me feel that way. I actually "become" what he sees.

That's the nicest part. And I believe in him.

Maybe that's what love is.

AUGUST 10

After Francine had us "talk" to the food in my new summer bulimia support group, I felt both a sense of strength and weakness, a feeling of exhilaration and anxiety. My first feelings were the positive ones. I had been so busy the past few weeks that I really hadn't been as obsessed with my "progress." Talking to the food made me realize that I had changed positively without even forcing myself. That's new because in the past I've felt as if I had to be controlling everything or else it wouldn't work. Here it was working without my conscious attention. Those were my immediate feelings. The next day, I started to question myself. "Where do you come off thinking that you're doing okay? Stop kidding yourself. You've just been too busy to eat." That day I was hot and tired and thought I was getting sick, and I overate. But without forcing myself to stop, I just did—without finishing what I had bought and for no reason except that I didn't like the way it was physically making me feel—and I just didn't want it.

Although I haven't been seeing Francine every week since Dad recently angrily cut off my one-on-one therapy, going to her group twice a month is a good way to reflect on what's been happening (and a lot cheaper).

All in all, talking to the food showed me that while I may have a grip on my problem, my grip may still be too tight. I've got to let myself breathe.

AUGUST 17

Well, Bob arrived early, and what an arrival.

Friends for our whole freshman year. The closest of friends and nothing happens.

He's back one day and BOOM!

When he got up to close the door of his apartment after it had been open all day, and he came over to the couch and sat very close to me and stared at me, my heart almost stopped beating I got so scared.

This was after, for the first time, we talked about our prospective love lives. He's met Perry, but we've *never* talked about it. He started mentioning his girlfriend in Wisconsin. GIRLFRIEND! I saw one picture once in his apartment shortly after we met and then it was gone.

So, I told him about how Perry and I aren't really seeing each other anymore and mainly about Brent and David, a new person I had met at a work party who was sending me flowers and asking me out every weekend.

I told him how I was disappointed in what I'd seen in Brent. Here we were, flirting friends at the TV studio for a year, thinking we'd be really good together, all the right components, and we finally "date" for a few weeks and . . . It was very easy for me to see quickly a relationship with Brent would not be for me. Talent, charisma, chutzpah, but what underneath? I couldn't find anything for me. When I wanted to talk it was like he had to keep it light and funny. *Had to.* I don't want that.

And then Bob, who has never sat this close to me, says, "What did you think of me all last year?"

"I guess I thought you weren't interested."

"Weren't interested? After you moved off campus, you were never around. Never came around. I love you and I have for a long time."

That's what everyone had said. Noreen. Mom. Everyone who had seen us together said, "Don't you see the way he looks at you?" But I didn't.

And I said, "I love you, too."

I thought of last year at Christmas break when I took him to the airport and we held hands to run to the terminal and I wished it were real. This Christmas, I can kiss him goodbye, and I'll be his girlfriend, and I didn't even have to wait until Christmas either.

AUGUST 17

The urge to eat is so strong whenever I feel as though I've overeaten, even by a little. And yet, this is so illogical. If eating is the problem, then why eat to appease the problem? Maybe for a while I can't trust my body urges. They've been trained to work against me. Just because my body says, do this, do that, doesn't mean I have to listen.

I'm tired of working against myself in the guise of working for myself. It's ridiculous. It's a circle that I get lost in. I get so concerned with staying on that fine line that *is* the circle. If I take a step in, I'll fall in. If I take a step out, I'll fall out. Or so I think. Maybe there's really land on both sides of the circle, and, if I step off, I'll realize I don't have to spend all that energy balancing.

AUGUST 20

From a page working deep inside a television soundstage:

Dear Perry,

I'm only writing because I'm so busy, I'll probably be home for a total of two minutes in the next three days. This will probably reach you before I could even call. I tried to call you today from work, but you weren't home.

I've been thinking, I don't like the way we (I) left things after we talked the other night. You're right, I don't want you out of my life. We *are* friends. Finally, because I'm not exactly sure what we were before. After we talked on the phone, I realized how far we've both come. We are different than we were, so how can we know how we feel? We can't. After I talked to you I thought, who can I talk to like this, this openly, about anything and everything, without being uncomfortable, even after not seeing each other for four months? This *is* special.

You're right. I was trying to tie everything up in a little package. And, of course, it can't be done. I did the same thing that I used to do: It had to be all or nothing. Which is ridiculous, since I don't even know what "it all" is, let alone if I want it. What I see now is that I don't want nothing, either.

I am your friend. I do want to see you. I don't want to cut you out of my life, and I'm glad that you don't want to cut me out of yours. So, instead of saying good-bye and good luck, I'll say, keep in touch.

Love,
Lisa

Seeking Help for Yourself or Someone You Care About

If you are one of the millions like Lisa, at this point, you are now more aware of what has been happening to you. You realize that the eating disorder, to a very great extent, has taken over your life. You are no longer in control. You also have realized that self-treatment is not possible and that this journey is one that cannot, and does not need to be, made alone. You have made the decision to seek help.

In this chapter, I will focus on how to seek help and what that help can do for you. We will look at how to begin, and what an ideal outpatient treatment team should look like. I will briefly explore what various professionals can do and what to expect from each member of a therapeutic team so that you can make the best possible and most informed choices. We will also look at when inpatient treatment is the best choice and what you can expect in an inpatient setting.

You are about to embark on one of the most significant journeys of your life. At times, the road will be smooth, but at other times you may feel that you are on a roller coaster, as, like Lisa, you seem to make progress and then slide back. Do not be discouraged. Moving backward and forward—relapses—are to be expected. At times the road will be longer than you had expected. Remember, there is hope. You can overcome your eating disorder, regaining control of your body and of your life.

Even more importantly, you are no longer alone. You are securing a vital support network of friends, family, and skilled professionals. Lisa will also be accompanying you on the road to recovery as you share her roller coaster ride, as the challenges she faces may mirror your own. Some of her struggles will be very familiar to you and others may be different than what you are experiencing, as each individual is unique. All will help you to better understand what may initially be a frightening and confusing time, as you begin to grow and change.

WHERE TO BEGIN

As simple as it sounds, the first place to begin is to tell someone what is happening. You have probably kept your eating disorder a closely guarded secret for all of the reasons we have already described. It is now essential to break that veil of secrecy and come out of your isolation. If you are a teenager or young adult, you can begin by telling a family member or a close and trusted friend, but it is important to also let an adult know what is occurring. Lisa told her mother and did not tell her father until much later. The choice of who to tell is yours, but you must tell someone. Lisa ended up finding her own psychological help and that therapist then became the person she confided in about her previous secret behavior.

When you decide from whom you will seek support, find a quiet place and time and explain what you are experiencing. He or she cannot only help you find the help you need, but also perhaps continue to be there as a support in the months to come. Whatever your age, speaking to a family member, your doctor, a trusted friend, or a religious leader will break your isolation and most likely start you on a helpful path. A benefit of speaking to your doctor either first or as soon as posible will be the immediate ability to assess the sometimes extensive physical damage caused by your eating disorder, beginning with the proper diagnosis and treatment of your physical body. That is only the beginning. If possible, it is important to see a doctor who has had previous experience with eating disorders. Most family doctors are knowledgeable about eating disorders and may provide important referrals to other professionals. If your doctor has limited knowledge about eating disorders, however, help him or her to better understand the severity of what you are experiencing (as Lisa did with her father) and the need for a complete physical checkup.

Talking to someone who has previously been or is currently in treatment can be useful, although it is important to remember that each journey has unique parts. If you know someone who has been through it, ask her what she has done to seek help. If she is willing, ask her to share the names of the professionals she has found helpful and information about how to reach those professionals. The name of a professional who has been successful in helping a friend can be invaluable, and you will probably find your friend not only more than willing to share resources, but also very supportive of your decision. If you know no one who has been in treatment, consider using the Internet for resources. There are so many sites that can provide useful information as well as referrals. Some places to start with might include IAEDP (International Association of Eating Disorder Professionals), NEDA (National Eating Disorder Association), and Something Fishy. This list is only a very partial beginning. Please see the Resource List on page 237 for more information.

Attending an Overeaters Anonymous (OA) meeting also can be invaluable. Most of you will be able to find an OA meeting in your home area. Depending on your location, other support groups may also be available. In these meetings, you will most certainly find that you are not alone, and that there are so many others who understand and have experienced what you are going through. In addition, members can be a useful source of information about local professionals and programs that they have found helpful. Finally, OA members can provide enormous support and often long-term friendships. Although certain basic structures and concepts can be found in each group, memberships differ. It may be useful to try more than one group to find out where you are most comfortable, as trust and openness will be key parts of your OA success, as well as the success of the other parts of your program.

YOUR TREATMENT TEAM

Seeking help means gathering a team of professionals that are there to support and guide you in your recovery. This team, without question, should include a physician and psychotherapist or counselor. Nutritionists and dentists are also vital to a full recovery. But don't worry—you're not expected to seek out every team member all at once. This is the ideal comprehensive plan. Focus on contacting your doctor or psychologist first, who then can provide referrals for others who will be there to help you. Let's explore what you can expect from each.

Primary Care Physician

The first person you should see is either your primary care physician or your new psychotherapist, psychologist, or psychiatrist. If possible, start with the primary care physician, your family doctor. If it is difficult to talk about what is going on to your doctor, take a trusted friend with you for support. You will probably find that your doctor is caring, sympathetic, and professional. In addition, if you have been seeing the doctor for a period of time, he or she will have a baseline of what normal health is for you. This can be very useful, because you want to chart what has been your unique normal health in the past against what is currently occurring.

It is normal to be nervous during the visit and you may forget some very important things. It may also have been a long time since you talked about your physical body to anyone. Therefore, beforehand, write down all of the physical problems you are aware of, as well as any strange feelings or unusual things you are experiencing in your body or any physical symptoms that are different than the norm. Do not think that anything you write is silly, trivial, or embarrassing. All are parts of the puzzle that you and your doctor will attempt to put together.

The medical visit will have three major purposes. First, it will determine whether there are any other physical reasons for the symptoms you are having. Second, it will assess the impact of your illness on your current health. Third, it will determine whether any more serious steps need to be taken medically. During the visit, what will occur is a check of your current weight. Lab work will probably include blood work, checking vitamin and mineral levels, white blood cells, glucose and electrolyte levels, and cholesterol levels. A complete CBC as well as a complete metabolic profile are standard. Your doctor will want to check for menstrual irregularities, blood pressure problems, and heart rhythms. A thyroid screening is frequently done, as well as a serum magnesium and urinalysis. If you are 15 percent or more below normal body weight, a chest x-ray and other tests (like complement3, 24creatinine clearance, uric acid, and testing for high catacolamines) may be performed.

Share with your doctor the list of common physical symptoms of eating disorders that I listed in *How to Identify an Eating Disorder*. This may seem like overkill, but remember, what is at stake is your life! If your doctor has limited knowledge about eating disorders, help him or her to better understand the severity of what you are experiencing and the need for a complete physical checkup. You are your best advocate. If you do not have a regular doctor, ask a friend for a recommendation. If you are at college, go to the school health center. Go to the Internet, beginning with the sources we have already listed, to see if knowledgeable physicians in your home area are listed. The American Medical Association can also provide lists of doctors in your geographic area, although there is no certainty these doctors are skilled in treating eating disorders.

Therapist

The most important person accompanying you on your journey will probably be your psychotherapist, psychologist, or psychiatrist. Lisa worked with both an individual and a group psychotherapist. Ideally, he or she will be with you for the length of your treatment, and can also help you access skilled and qualified professionals to complete the treatment team. Formally, he or she will help you unwrap and control the eating disorder symptoms that are so troubling, as we have seen firsthand happening with Lisa. More importantly, your therapist will help you to understand the underlying issues that are at the root of your eating disorder symptoms, causing the disorder and continuing to maintain it. He or she will help you to explore what is happening inside you as well as what is happening around you, such as your family dynamics, friendships, school and work pressures—all of the things that make you uniquely you. In the process, like Lisa, you will be surprised at your new insights, as you find out more and more about a very important person—you! Finally, your therapist will work with you on your steps to recovery, developing new understandings and finding coping skills that no longer center on body image, food, and exercise.

This is what will formally occur. Although the therapy may sometimes feel difficult, you may be relieved to find comfort in someone to lean on who really understands. Informally, your therapist may become a trusted mentor, teacher, friend, spiritual guide, and anchor in the sometimes-stormy path to come.

Your therapist can be a licensed psychologist, psychiatrist, social worker, mental health counselor, or addictions professional. The most important criteria are his or her training and expertise in the field of eating disorders. What is equally important is the relationship that you develop with your therapist. As we witnessed with Lisa, she did not feel comfortable with the older male therapist her mother's doctor recommended, but felt immediately at ease with the young female therapist she found through an ad in the university newspaper. Experience and expertise in the field of eating disorders is very important, but relationship is key. It is essential to feel that your therapist hears you, understands and can interpret, and offers advice that makes sense to you. If you do not respect and trust your therapist, opening up will be difficult.

Give the relationship time to develop. After all, you have become adept at keeping secrets. It may have been a long time since you completely and fully trusted and really felt anyone could help. This, like other important relationships, may take some time to form. Try to be as open and honest with your thoughts and feelings as you can be. In the therapy sessions, you can talk about anything. You will not be judged. Don't be afraid to ask for what you need, and, if you feel you are not being heard or understood, let your therapist know. If you still feel the therapy is not helping, consider a consultation with another therapist who will help you figure out whether this is the right therapist for you.

Lisa found her therapist by reading about her in the college newspaper, and she entered a separate group therapy at the university. If you are on a college campus, your health or counseling centers may be able to help you find the right therapist. Most have eating-disorders professionals on staff and many have ongoing eating disorder programs. If you are in high school, your guidance counselor may be able to help. Overeaters Anonymous can provide resources, a friend with an eating disorder can help locate a therapist, and the organizations listed above (and in the Resource List) can provide names of qualified professionals in your area.

Psychiatrist

The psychiatrist can play multiple roles in the treatment of an eating disorder. In some treatment centers, the psychiatrist is the head of the treatment team or medical director of the eating disorder program. The psychiatrist may also serve as the primary therapist, although this is usually the role of the psychologist, social worker, or eating-disorders counselor.

In all cases, the psychiatrist evaluates for and prescribes psychotropic medication, when it is deemed necessary. These medications may not only aid in the reduction of current symptoms, but also aid in the prevention of relapse. Equally important, these medications treat the co-morbidities (associated medical illnesses) such as depression, anxiety, mood disorders, personality disorders, and addictions. Frequently used medications include Prozac, Paxil, Zoloft, Remeron, SSRI's, and mood stabilizers like Depakote. There are two points that are important to bear in mind. First and foremost, all medication must be prescribed and monitored by a skilled psychiatrist. Second, if used, medication is only a part of the treatment approach, and medication alone will rarely lead to long-term recovery.

Group Psychotherapist

Under the guidance of a skilled group therapist, groups can provide an important adjunct to individual therapy. The group can be a source of information, support, education, empowerment, motivation, and hope. The group can help to provide a safety net when so many things around you feel unsafe. Along with individual therapy, group therapy can aid you in discovering and exploring the underlying issues involved in your eating disorder, thereby helping you to find answers and solutions.

For many, the feeling that no one else could ever fully understand has been a powerful one for a long time. In the group, you will find that there are others who truly understand and have shared parts of your journey. This feeling, called universality, will be a powerful force in helping you move out of your self-imposed isolation, as you learn to share and lean on others again. At the same time, you will be an important force in helping others to grow. You will not only be receiving help but giving help, and within this giving, strong friendships are often forged, as group members continue the journey back to health together.

For Lisa, group psychotherapy was an important part of her growth. When group ended for the summer, she felt sadness and loss. Her letters to fellow group member Jane served as an outlet, support, and safety net during the summer months. "Your letter was a relief," Lisa wrote. "Really. I felt like I was reading something that I could have written. Finally, I thought, someone who understands, and who I understand!" The letters also served to provide additional insights. "Things here have not gone well, but I'm reacting and showing my feelings and weaknesses instead of pigging out," Jane wrote. "Knowing that I can handle stressful situations and not fall apart has made me like myself so much more." Lisa writes back about her changing relationship with food, her boyfriends, renewing old friendships, and her increasing insights about her father. Later, Jane shares another important insight," About the family problems I mentioned in my last letter, I decided in the midst of all this that I could either take all the problems upon myself and go bananas, or I could love, support, and be concerned but not let it get to me. . . . It really is more like self-respect and self-love." And so the group continues through the summer in the form of the true friendship Lisa and Jane have formed. More importantly, Lisa has moved out of a position of secrecy and isolation and has risked sharing her deepest and most personal feelings in written form, not only to her diary, but also to a real person.

Nutritionist

I cannot stress enough the importance of having a nutritionist (if possible) as a part of your treatment team. When this is not possible, your therapist will often be placed in the position of playing a multiple role for which he or she may not be trained and which can hamper the therapy process. As you already know, changing your relationship with food is a key to therapeutic success.

The first step is finding a nutritionist who is well-versed in the treatment of eating disorders. Lisa saw a nutritionist prior to admitting to anyone she had an eating disorder, theoretically, to lose some weight, even though she was not overweight. The nutritionist gave her a moderate-calorie eating plan, which Lisa then secretly slashed to fewer calories to further limit her food intake and sink more and more into her eating disorder. Even though the nutritionist was treating some eating-disordered patients (especially anorectics) as well as weight-loss clients, she did not recognize Lisa's problem and congratulated Lisa on her successful weight loss (from 128 pounds to 116 pounds, as a 5'4" 16 year old). Lisa continued to severely restrict herself with the food plans that stemmed from the nutritionist (whom she had only seen for a few months) for years after she stopped seeing the nutritionist. And when Lisa returned to the nutritionist as a 112-pound 18 year old who had starved herself to that weight and was trying desperately not to regain weight, the nutritionist asked her why she needed to be there since she looked so great.

The problem: This nutritionist probably had little experience in treating eating disorders. Your eating-disorders-trained nutritionist will not be there primarily to give you a meal plan, although that may be a small part of the overall picture. She will also *not* be there to make you gain weight. That is important to realize. Let's look at what may happen when you visit a nutritionist who specializes in the treatment of eating disorders.

Your nutritionist will probably begin by assessing your current eating patterns and nutritional intake. Try to be as honest as possible, even though it may not be easy to talk about what you have or have not been eating. Again, as with your therapist, you will be speaking to a neutral and interested listener and you will not be judged. During this initial assessment period, the nutritionist will be collecting data not only about your food intake, but also about your relationship with food. It is also during this period that you will be establishing a rapport or relationship with your nutritionist. It is this comfort level and relationship that will be essential in allowing you to examine the important role of food in your life and to begin to change some ingrained ideas and concepts about your previous best friend and worst enemy. Lisa told me that, unlike with her future therapist, whenever she was around the young woman who was her nutritionist, she felt guarded and like she was being judged and had to be a "good," "perfect" girl in following the meal plan. You must feel comfortable with your nutritionist.

Your nutritionist will also be a teacher. He or she will work to educate you about normal eating patterns and about the physiologic and metabolic consequences of normal and abnormal eating, helping you to become more aware of your own body as well as helping you to understand the significant consequences of your current eating patterns. It is here that comfort and relationship are vital, because if no relationship has developed, you will either not hear or tend to disregard what is being said. What will, in effect, be happening is a form of reparenting as your previously held misconceptions about food and weight are explored and challenged, and as you gain new awareness and perspectives on your body and on food.

It is during this phase that you will be supported in making incremental changes towards normalized eating. In addition, you may have become detached from your body and no longer have the ability to know when you are full—that is, you are not aware of somatic hunger and satiety sensations. A nutritionist well-versed in the issues of eating disorders can help you get back in touch with your body and learn about satiety so that you can again know when your body is telling you it has had enough food. In brief, you will learn again to trust your body cues.

Your nutritionist as well as your therapist will help you to understand the connection between emotions, food, and body image behaviors. You will learn about the foods that trigger a binge. You will also learn about the emotions and body image distortions that trigger a binge, exercise bulimia, bulimia, or starvation behavior. Some of this work will be done with your nutritionist and some with your psychotherapist, as this is an area of overlap. You will be continuing to explore the fact that this is not about food, but about the other issues that trigger the food response and the steps necessary for change.

Practically, you will be aided in finding a "good" weight for yourself. You, with the aid of your nutritionist, will decide the weight range you want to achieve. It is at this stage that a food plan may be suggested, helping you get to and maintain the chosen weight as you learn to practice positive weight maintenance. This part of the journey is not always an easy one, as you may find yourself changing not only previously held concepts and beliefs, but also ingrained habits. Your nutritionist will be there to support, encourage, and, when necessary, implement changes as you find, probably to your surprise, that your new plan works. You may also find that your new relationship with food can be fun. Some nutritionists take you shopping to new places to explore variety in food choices. Others may assist you in eating-out behavior as you again experiment with a new and growing variety of choices. Some nutritionists will give you new recipes and novel ways to prepare food within the calorie range you have chosen together. All will be working to assure that food is no longer the enemy.

Dentist

Physical changes in the mouth are often the first signs of an eating disorder. All eating disorders can cause dry mouth, swollen salivary glands, and lips that are red, dry, or cracked. Nutritional deficits can have serious dental consequences. Anorexia can cause saliva deficiencies in the buffers that protect teeth from the effects of acids manufactured by the bacteria in the mouth—and many low-calorie drinks and diet sodas contain significant acid. Normal saliva, which helps protect teeth from acid, makes its buffers in part from materials found in fatty foods, which may have been severely limited as part of the eating disorder.

Bulimia can have far more serious effects on dental health. Repeated vomiting causes loss of tooth enamel. Teeth may become rounded and soft and may change in color, shape, and length. Fillings may start to rise above the tooth surface. Teeth can become brittle, translucent, and very sensitive to temperature changes. In more serious cases, the innermost layer of the tooth can become exposed, causing infection or death of the tooth. A visit to the dentist to assess the current state of your dental health, particularly if your eating disorder is bulimia, is important and something you may not have previously considered.

Coaching

The relatively new and growing field of coaching may be a useful adjunct to your treatment. However, in no cases should it be a substitute for ongoing psychotherapy. Caroline Miller, a well-respected coach, describes coaching as having someone with whom you can share your goal of overcoming your eating disorder and who can help you focus your energies most efficiently to achieve your goals. Most coaching is client centered and so you will set the agenda, largely direct the process, and provide most of the material for the work. The coach will guide, direct, support, and encourage.

Caroline describes some of the goals many people work toward as the following: working on assertiveness skills; developing a workable, noncompulsive fitness plan; learning to prioritize; assembling health care professionals and friends who are supportive; envisioning fears that prevent success; identifying other addictions; and achieving financial independence. One of the advantages of coaching is that it can be done from the home or workplace, on the telephone, or over the Internet. Also, some of the coaches, like Caroline, have recovered from an eating disorder and can completely understand you—and are able to share techniques and treatments they have found effective in their own recovery. Finally, they can serve not only as teacher and mentor but as a model, showing that you, too, can achieve long-term recovery.

Inpatient Treatment

Inpatient treatment means staying at a hospital or residential treatment center for a period of time. All of what I have been discussing thus far has had to do with outpatient treatment. What that means is that you continue living where and how you have been living and seek an independent therapist or treatment team. Sometimes outpatient treatment is just not enough and residential treatment becomes the only choice. The decision to enter inpatient treatment is sometimes completely clear, but, at other times, the choice is a difficult one. A basic rule of thumb: The greater the problem, the more need to manage it intensively. If you are in medical crisis, if your quality of life is so compromised that you feel you cannot go on, or if outpatient treatment will not work or is not working, then inpatient treatment might be your best choice. What else would be useful to know in making this important decision?

Although Lisa lost weight and her exercise-starvation dieting bulimia and binge eating reached significant proportions, she was one of the lucky ones. Medically, she never reached crisis stage. Even though most of you are thinking, yes, that's me, too, a large percentage of you will not actually be so lucky. Your medical symptoms can very rapidly reach serious or even critical proportions. Medical crisis is a clear indicator that inpatient treatment is necessary. Teens with eating disorders are particularly at risk, but medical necessity can come unexpectedly at any age.

Indicators of medical instability that may require hospitalization include: hypothermia, severe bradycardia (heartbeat 45 beats per minute or below), hypotension or shock, severe malnutrition (defined as less than 75 percent of normal body weight), arrested growth or development, acute food refusal, electrolyte imbalance, uncontrollable binging and purging, other acute medical symptoms or an acute psychiatric emergency, including suicidal thoughts or psychotic thoughts, and a failure to respond to outpatient treatment. Some inpatient treatment centers are equipped to deal with acute medical emergencies. Many are not. If you are in severe medical crisis (your family doctor can help you make that determination), a short hospital stay before inpatient treatment may be necessary to stabilize your health before entering inpatient treatment.

The length of time of inpatient treatment may vary widely from a few days to a few months. The length depends on the severity of your eating disorder and your response to treatment. Unfortunately, inpatient treatment can be very costly and your length of stay may also be determined in part by your insurance coverage. The treatment center that you choose can help you determine medical benefits and can often contact and negotiate with your insurance company.

Who will be your inpatient treatment team? At many of the centers around the country, your treatment team may include your primary therapist, who will usually be a psychologist or social worker; psychiatrist; family therapist; nutritionist; physicians; nurses; art and movement therapists; and an aftercare counselor who will be essential in your transition home, in aftercare preparation, and in relapse prevention. Treatment modalities vary widely. All will include talk therapy, which may be psychodynamic, behavioral, cognitive, humanistic, gestalt, interpersonal, psychodramatic, or systems oriented. All have the same goal—relief from symptoms and work on the underlying issues leading to and perpetuating your eating disorder—as well as long-term health. Some centers will incorporate movement, art, psychodrama, music, equine therapy, and spirituality work.

Since programs vary widely, it is important to be an educated consumer. Whenever possible, find out what you can about the treatment center. Ask about the average length of stay and the success rate. Find out the programs and treatment offered and what part is done individually and what part in group therapy. Is there a family therapy component? Is the program a large or small one? Frequently, the larger programs can offer a wider variety of services, while the smaller programs are more individually oriented, although this is not always the case. Does the program have a religious or spiritual orientation? Are there other people your age in the program (particularly important for younger children and teenagers)? Is a medical doctor available (key if medical stability is an issue)? Will you have an individual psychotherapist? Will you be educated in relapse prevention? Will the facility help you to establish an aftercare program and aid in your transition back into the community? Finally, and unfortunately important, will the facility work with you in gaining insurance coverage? National Association of Anorexia Nervosa and Associated Disorders (ANAD) can also be contacted directly with questions and concerns about insurance. See the Resource List on page 237 for more information.

Sometimes it is possible to visit the program and observe. Never be afraid to ask questions. The treatment center that you choose will be important, but you and you alone will provide the key to your successful treatment. Your hard work in getting better and your success in treatment will truly be something that you can control.

Although treatment centers vary, all work to alleviate the symptoms of your eating disorder and address the psychological and environmental issues that are at the root of your disorder. The well-respected Renfrew Center's four-stage program is a good example of what you might expect. Stage One is a time for stabilization in which you will work to eliminate the immediate physical and emotional dangers of your eating disorder. In this stage, you will begin to gain an increased sense of safety and control. Stage Two has to do with symptom management. During this stage, you will work intensively to understand and confront the underlying issues of your disorder. You will also begin to develop lifetime coping skills, learning to control destructive behaviors. As you have seen with Lisa, eating disorders are a persistent illness and cure is not rapid. Most likely, you will move forward and slide back, as Lisa did. She felt confusion at times. She gained and lost weight, but she never again felt trapped in all of those rules and obsessions. However, everyone's story is unique, and, for many, difficulties with food, weight, and exercise may reemerge unexpectedly for a long time, sometimes for many years.

In Stage Three you will learn relapse prevention. You will work on developing a healthy relationship with food and will learn practical skills to maintain your physical and emotional health for the rest of your life. You will also learn that relapses can happen and what to do when they occur. Stage Four varies widely from center to center. At many centers you may return to school or work during the day and return for continuing treatment each evening. At other centers, inpatient treatment continues with fewer hours of therapy. You will be transitioning back into normal life and into your outpatient treatment. It is important that this treatment be set up in advance so that the transition is a smooth one, as you may be returning to many of the pressures of your old life. However, you probably will have grown and learned. You are probably more aware and healthier. Therefore, you will probably lean on others when necessary, and with continuing support, you will handle them differently.

Perhaps most importantly, the centers likely will provide a warm, caring, and supportive atmosphere. You will feel safe to risk and to change. You may feel a freedom that you have not felt for a very long time. You will learn a tremendous amount about your eating disorder. You will learn a tremendous amount about your life, your family and, most importantly, yourself.

I hope you now realize the importance of seeking help, and will be enriched through the process of self-discovery that comes through therapy. The knowledge and insights you gain from your treatment team professionals will teach you so much about yourself and will undoubtedly be important for the rest of your life, and, in fact, in my final chapter we'll talk about just that: advice to live the rest of your life healthfully in the real world. First, let's take a firsthand look at how Lisa negotiates that real world as she moves further and further away from her eating disorder.

11. Love Affair
19 TO 21 YEARS OLD

I feel trapped. Now that I'm controlling my weight, it's okay to binge again. I realize that this was the problem to begin with, binging as a response to stress and other problems, and then watching very carefully what I ate (if anything) the following days. So, I feel like I'm getting trapped in that cycle again because for most of my life this cycle (and not crucial weight gain) has been my problem. Last year, I binged and didn't watch what I ate the following days, and I gained weight. Then, this past summer, I didn't binge at all, and ate, to some extent normally, and lost most of the weight. Now that the weight is not so bad (since I can leave the house and function socially, which I couldn't do when I was ten pounds heavier) I've been binging and then regulating again.

A few weeks ago, right before the first "old time" supermarket candy-cookie-cake-binge, my mind was saying, this is going to be comfortable. It was yearning for that old soothed feeling. Those actions and that feeling seemed a part of me, and, afterwards, it did seem like the normal thing for me to have done. It gave me that comfortable, soothed feeling.

I've also been binging when I feel I don't have control over my time. "Okay, so I've got to stay at school for hours between classes since I have to live so far away, but I'm staying under protest." "Okay, so I've got to take this traffic and go to my parents' home, where I'm not sure I want to be, I'll do that under protest, too," which means eating.

Of course, I don't *have* to live at home, but I haven't even brought up moving. My parents said I could if I want to. I am punishing myself. Who should lay out money for someone who almost dropped out again, who runs away from apartments? I want to prove myself first.

I can see another part of this whole thing, too. I haven't been having any fun. I haven't been giving myself anything. The thing is I can't think of anything I would like to do or buy or give myself that would make me feel good, and I don't know why. I have been going out, but now it's with David, someone with whom there seems to be strings attached. He's so intense. Flowers. Cards. It's still something that I want to do, but it's not always fun. Since he's been out of school for two years and already works in the entertainment law industry, he can't always relate to what I'm going through with school or my parents.

I can't help feeling that I am going out with him because Bob hurt me so much. I couldn't believe it. After so long, being so close, it comes down to this. The girl doesn't go to bed with me one-two-three, I drop her. Where is the sensitive person I've known, the one who said he loved me? Little did he know, because of the way I felt about him and feel, I was already planning a trip to the university's birth control clinic. I was floating on a cloud. He stuck a pin in the way I'm looking at everything. I was ready, not one-two-three, but I was ready. With him.

Another part of what I've been feeling is that if I don't get it now, I won't get it, at least at my parents' house. If there's cake or frozen pizza or corn chips, they won't last and they're not usually there. So I feel that I have to have it in the mornings that I don't have to leave for school at the crack of dawn. It is as though I'm giving myself something. This is my only do-nothing-but-relax time when no one else is around, and I spend it eating and reading the newspaper or eating and watching television. I don't feel guilty anymore, I don't really care if my family knows I ate it, but I still wouldn't eat it in front of them.

I've been feeling the whole thing is abnormal. My mind is saying that the only way I could conceive of really having fun, enjoying my free time or enjoying most people, is to be thin. I can see it now. My mind is saying that, although I weigh about 124 pounds, I can't truly be happy without weighing 110 or 114 pounds. Another part of me is saying that I don't want to be happy just *because* of that. So, I'm trapped in between and I'm eating. Then I think, what if I stopped binging and just ate normally and stayed where I am weight-wise? I know I am just afraid, afraid that I'll see the way it should be and *relax* for once in my life and stop striving. I'm afraid of this, but I'm not sure why.

SEPTEMBER 23

I gained five pounds in the last two days. Monday, I weighed 122. Thursday, I weigh at least $127\frac{1}{2}$.

Yesterday, I ate:
- 2 little pizzas
- 1 barrel of caramel corn with nuts
- 1 bag of cheese popcorn
- 1 bag of candy peanuts
- 2 hot dogs with mayonnaise
- 1 in a tortilla
- 1 in bread
- 1 frozen pancake breakfast
- 2 cans of Coke

And maybe more.

Tuesday, I ate:
- 1 frozen pancake breakfast
- *a lot* of Fritos
- 2 pieces of fudge
- 1 big cookie
- 1 piece of fruitcake

Late at night:
- 1 fast-food chicken sandwich
- 1 large French fries

Revelation 278:

I'm not weak because I decided to have dinner. I am stronger as a result of that somewhat balanced meal. Now, I have the energy to work on my essay.

WALK, WALK, WALK:
THAT'S ALL THE STUDENTS DO HERE

By Lisa Messinger

During the first week of school, I was rear-ended twice, side-swiped seven times, had three head-on collisions, and was the victim of a hit-and-run accident.

But don't be fooled, I have a perfect driving record, and there's not a scratch or a dent on my car. Rather it's my body that's been scratched and dented not to mention bumped, bruised, and mangled.

Lying in my recovery bed, I have come to the following conclusion: While it may not yet have been proven to cause cancer in laboratory rats, walking can definitely be hazardous to your health. At USC, that is.

Being a pedestrian is an experience unique unto itself. At first glance, it appears that the greatest perpetrators of the accidents I mentioned would be daydreaming bicyclists or tired tram drivers. Not true. Surprisingly, the gravest threat to our safety, not to mention sanity, is us. We've been stepping, trampling and stampeding all over each other.

Why? It's simple. We USC pedestrians are busy people. There aren't enough hours in a day to do our walking at one time and everything else we have to do at another time. Thus we combine the two. We walk and read. We walk and eat. We walk and talk. Boy, do we ever walk and talk.

Since walking can become habitual, rhythmic, automatic, and even boring, it entices us to attempt more difficult tasks simultaneously. Unfortunately, these other tasks drain concentration that is needed for walking. Just yesterday in the University Avenue/ Tommy Trojan vicinity I noticed an example of this problem. A fraternity pledge engrossed in *Playboy* ran down a sorority pledge engrossed in *Playgirl*. While it could have been love at first sight, we'll probably never know since they were knocked unconscious and are now in comas at County-USC Hospital.

Seconds after the paramedics carried them away, another mishap occurred. A pre-med student who was trying to jog to class, eat a taco salad, and dissect a frog all at the same time tripped and caused a ten-Trojan pileup in front of the music building.

Clearly something must be done. I have an idea. But I'm afraid that to some the idea may seem too severe, too harsh. Nevertheless, sometimes drastic measures are called for: Try watching where you are going.

Lisa Messinger is a sophomore majoring in broadcast journalism.

FREELOADER IN PINK BOXERS OVERSTEPS HIS BOUNDS

By Lisa Messinger

There's a guy living in my apartment. He's not my boyfriend, husband, brother, or friend. In fact, I know relatively nothing about him. What I do know is that he eats my food, copies my lecture notes, watches my TV, listens to my stereo, ties up my phone. And pays no rent.

You'd think he could be evicted, but, unfortunately, he can't. You see, he's not really a tenant. He's a freeloader, a pest, and an annoyance. In other words, he's my roommate's boyfriend.

And until the other day, I was putting up with his little idiosyncrasies. That was until he overstepped the bounds of peaceful co-existence. First, he had the nerve to ask for his own keys. He wanted both a door key and a mailbox key, since his mail is now being forwarded to our address.

Next, he asked if I would be kind enough to knock before entering the apartment. He said he was just being considerate since he knew it embarrassed me to find him watching TV in his underwear. Coincidentally, as he was making these requests, he was sprawled on the couch in nothing but a pair of pink polka-dot boxer shorts. I thanked him for his consideration of my feelings and told him that pink was definitely his color.

Then I went into my own room to find his entomology project, a live termite collection, gnawing away at my bedpost. They had gotten out of their cigar box.

At that point, I would have given anything if my roommate's boyfriend would have gotten out of our apartment.

It was then and there that I knew I had had enough. Being able to think of no other options, I went with the honest approach. I went out to the kitchen to find him at the freezer eyeing my Haagen-Dazs ice cream. Quite simply, I told him to pack up his termites and never to show his spotted boxer shorts at my doorstep again. It worked. He and my roommate moved out that same night. They're now residing at his place.

Sorry, Arnold. (That's *his* roommate.)

Lisa Messinger is a sophomore majoring in broadcast journalism.

[Made up as a good topic of a humor column, since I was then living at my parents' house. Based on when I was living with the roommate I didn't like.]

NOVEMBER 2

I did an experiment. I decided to live my life as an ordinary person. Average. Instead of above average. That's because although I am not ugly or fat, I don't feel pretty or thin either. I'm in between. I don't stand out in either direction anymore. I'm just there. Blah. Ick. Not awful. But nothing. Overreaction? Maybe. I can't tell.

It felt right to feel sick again over food. Like, welcome home. Comfortable. Like I've been away for a long time, but come back to the warmth, the numbness. Come back to where it doesn't hurt (on the surface) anymore. Come back. Come back. Come back.

NOVEMBER 3

Wheels are in motion. I feel alive again. I didn't even realize that I didn't before I left home to stay with my slightly younger cousin Vicki since her mom was going out of town on a long business trip. But I can see now I was feeling lifeless. Honestly, whenever I'd eat, I'd feel justified because I couldn't think of anything else that was more desirable. Nothing. And I couldn't understand why. Talking with any friends, going out with David, it just took on no meaning. With everything I had, I felt as though I had nothing. That's when I began to feel depressed, and as I said, I couldn't understand why.

Now that I've recognized I was feeling that way, I have some partial ideas as to why. I felt as though I was "doing," "putting out," and drawing nothing, no good feelings, from the people and things that made up my life.

I see now that risk is the only way you can really get in your corner the stuff you really want. Without it, you have to wait and wait and wait to be picked or chosen. Sometimes you're lucky. Those who pick and choose know what they want. Sometimes it's you, and sometimes, perhaps, you want them, too, but not usually as much as they want you. They've gotten what they really wanted. You got picked. They got the thrill of winning. You get to feel like the trophy. Well, I see now I want the thrill for myself. Sure, flattery is nice, but it wears off. I'll forego some of the flattery to do some of the picking.

That's why I felt such a rush from Brent and Bob. I didn't do it all, but I actively participated in the cultivation. I played a part in the desire process. Before I had them, I wanted each, consciously or subconsciously. That's the difference with David. He wants me, he loves me, he needs me, he picked me. I like him a great deal, but it's not the same thing. It's not the same rush, the same thrill of actively pursuing your life.

Now I've gotten that thrill with Greg. We had been close friends and more than friends for so long. Even just recently, he had told me how much he loved me; I think he meant as a person, as a close friend, but it felt good. And I had feelings and I finally felt free enough to express them now. I don't understand all of them, but I know they're there. He is inexplicably attractive to me on the physical and personality level, and I wanted him to know it, and I wanted to know he knew it, to know that I counted. I think we're beyond our "window," beyond the point of anything truly deep happening between us—and, besides, I'm dating David now—but these feelings needed to come out and I am relieved I finally expressed them.

NOVEMBER 12

No one has ever treated me as David does. He is so expressive. He is always telling me and showing me how he feels for me, making me feel special. And he's patient. He doesn't want me to do anything until I am ready.

I get to really, really like him more and more. I mean I liked him immediately. How many men do you see drinking Diet Pepsi at a party where everyone else is *drinking*? I had a feeling about him, and I was right. He had been heavy. Finally, I thought, maybe a man who will understand the desperation, loneliness, and insecurity I've been through.

And what do I get, a person never lonely or downtrodden, surrounded by *so many* friends. I have never met anyone with so many friends. He is so funny and outgoing and intelligent and has taken me under his wing.

We're becoming sidekicks, going everywhere together. It's not the kind of relationship I've gone for before, not that drop dead attraction (at least for me), but it's certainly the most comfortable I've ever felt with anyone. He makes me feel that way. I do believe he's madly in love with me, and that's awfully hard to resist.

NOVEMBER 14

Female wanted to take over housing contract in university housing as soon as possible. Call Penny: 213-555-2478.

* * * * *

Well, I got it. My own dorm room. No sharing. One of the only singles available. I think I'll like it. I can be around people and still have my privacy.

DECEMBER 12

The murderess trapped inside the expanded and uglied corpse. Forced to live everyday inside the mind of the beautiful girl she killed. Remembering. Remembering what it was like to be beautiful. Feeling. Feeling what it is like to be ugly. Knowing. Knowing she killed someone at the utmost prime of her life. A girl who looked and felt wonderful. A girl who had everything going for her and was going everywhere with everyone at once. That girl is dead, but she was never buried. She's rotting inside of the murderess. Rotting away, but not going away.

Every time the murderess sees someone who looks like the dead girl, she hates them on sight and isn't always sure why. She hates them more when the boy who was attracted to the dead girl is attracted to the look-alike and treats her like he used to treat the dead girl.

She doesn't hate the boy, though, just the look-alike. She understands the boy. He likes a pretty girl.

It's strange that the murderess hates herself, but loves the dead girl. The dead girl was the only girl she ever loved. The dead girl knew how to be happy without trying, without force. She just was. The murderess can't ever be happy. She could die if she could bring the dead girl back. But the dead girl is gone. And the murderess is trapped.

DECEMBER 13

12:43 A.M. *IN A ROOM OF MY OWN*
I just lost my virginity to one David Sorrell whom I love. Unexpectedly and unplanned I let him come inside of me. He's madly in love with me. I wanted it like crazy. And now I don't have to climb the walls anymore.

1:32 A.M.
It's 1:32 A.M. and he just left.

Well, I lost my virginity while I was still a teenager. Just barely. A month and a half until I'm twenty. I lost it when I was nineteen. But there's still more to learn and more to come.

DECEMBER 18

Friday, 2:41 A.M.
I feel like I just lost my virginity again. This time there really was no doubt about what was going on.

This all happened after a sitcom's TV wrap party. Funny, after the TV show wrap parties just a year ago, I was happy with a few kisses from my boyfriends. Not anymore.

DECEMBER 22

When I walked into Francine Snyder's office a few weeks ago, I talked to her about my feelings regarding the murderess and the happy beautiful thin girl. As it turned out, that was one of the last visits I made to Francine's office, because that was the day both the murderess and the illusion of the beautiful happy dead girl died.

The vision of a murderess had been brewing in my mind for a long time, ever since I gradually started gaining back the weight I had lost in the summer after my high school graduation. That was when for a few months I turned into the beautiful, happy, skinny, very popular girl I had always dreamed of being. It became etched in my mind with every pound that I gained that I was killing that girl, smothering her with chocolate syrup and malted milk balls.

Even through a year of bulimia counseling, although I have made incredible breakthroughs, I still clung to the idea of this beautiful happy thin girl who had proven to me that losing weight (as little as ten pounds) could in fact dramatically change your life. After all, I had been living proof of it!

What I finally realized that day in Francine's office as she had me role-play the part of the beautiful happy thin dead girl was that I had not really been happy then. I had been a robot, a beautiful, popular, skinny *robot*. I neither really thought nor felt during that time. I merely performed robot-like actions. My life had not been filled with the happiness I now chose to believe it had been filled with. Instead, it was filled, and completely saturated, with control, regimented diet, exercise, and even dating schedules. I wasn't free, I was like a machine.

That day was the first time I cried in her office because I realized there was no murderess. There was just me, the same girl who had inhabited my body before I invented that robot, the pretty girl who relied more on her brains than her looks. This was not a personality that I had "visualized" and then "achieved." This was a personality that was just, somehow, inexplicably there, as it had been before the weight loss.

That day, I felt a wave of self-acceptance come over me that was different from any other such feeling I had experienced while in therapy. Within weeks, I finally let myself fall into the love that had been building within me for David, who I'd already been seeing for almost four months. Also within weeks, I was able to do something I had been ready and wanting to do for some time, open myself up and give myself fully to another human being.

It would be nice to say that ever since that office visit and the consequential falling in love and loss of virginity that I have been contented and balanced. Well, I haven't been; everything's been more or less the same. It's just that I've had another realization, another very important realization.

DECEMBER 25

Sweetheart, when it comes to Christmas presents,
You're just what I've always wanted!
Merry Christmas, Sweetheart

I LOVE YOU
David

DECEMBER 30

Today:
- One "full" roast beef submarine sandwich
- One taco salad
- 6 macaroon bars
- 1 fast-food double burger
- 1 large French fries
- 1 large onion rings
- 1 medium chocolate shake

Plus regular diet breakfast and lunch

JANUARY 3

Vacationing in Palm Springs in Rented Condo With Family
I finally discovered that being happy is totally unrelated to weight or fluctuations of it, and I think it scared the hell out of me. After all, that's not the way I've been living for the past three or four or five years. It just crossed my mind a few minutes ago that I had been happy recently without the use of a scale.

My happy, elated sense of well-being really had nothing to do with weight or food. It had to do with feeling love and being loved and giving love and taking love in my relationship with David. In other words, it had to do with being free. And this freedom of just "being" is so new to me. I liked it. I got scared. And then I ate again.

But then I thought (after eating and eating), why am I eating? Then I ate some more. I had gotten so used to having my feelings come through food. Now it still brings me down quickly if I overeat a lot. It's not so much the actual eating (as it had been before), as it is the weight I feel I'm gaining from it. The main change has been with the rest of my eating. I don't have to follow rules and restrict my eating in order to feel good. I don't have to be an exact, certain weight, to feel good. Recently, I've pretty much just felt good, for no apparent reason, and with no strings attached.

Then, the past few days I've been progressively making myself feel bad, tearing myself down. The strange thing was that it didn't start because I felt fat. I didn't feel fat. I felt good. I felt I looked good, and not because of a scale number (I didn't know what it was), or because of eating too lightly (I wasn't restricting myself). I just felt good, I think, because I was letting myself be me and be free. I was doing for myself, and food and weight were not my main focus.

I was feeling nice without an incredible amount of trying, and now I'm feeling fat again. I feel like a seesaw, and that I can't trust or count on myself. Why would I want to take away an easy feeling of well-being to be miserable?

My eyes are tearing and my stomach is heaving because I had a sudden thought. Is it because then I am forced to go back into my old pattern? Yes. Yes. That's it. That's why today, especially, it seemed my interest was not in *what* I ate, but *that I keep eating* whenever my stomach could take anything. All day and night. I couldn't understand why I was doing that. It made me feel so much heavier that tomorrow I wanted to not eat anything—I felt boxed into that. Pushed onto the roller coaster.

But why would I do this? I like it the other way. No, I *love* it the other way, and now I feel so far removed from that other feeling that I have to struggle my way back. Because, of course, I can't stay the way I feel now.

LATER: I've discovered in the past few days with David here with me in Palm Springs that I like sex. I really like it. Maybe that's connected to the "stuffing" I've been doing. My feelings and actions in the past regarding sex have been pretty ambivalent. The past three weeks, the past few days, really, have been the first time I've ever truly let go, just feel, and listen to my body. (I didn't even know my body could tell me such things.)

A couple days ago, though, was the first time, I think, that I thought, "This feels so good. This *is* fun."

After so many boys had tried, the first time I was finally ever really involved in a kissing session—I was already over eighteen—Perry, my then boyfriend-to-be, pulled me back into his car (I was going to leave) and he said, "This is too much fun to stop." That struck me as very strange. Fun? No. No. No. This is serious business. It means things. It is something (I don't know what), but it is not (should not be) fun. I thought that through a year and a half of our relationship.

Then during this newer relationship with David, right from the beginning, I had a different attitude—an attitude that first said, you deserve this and then said, hey, this is okay. But I still couldn't just go with the flow. I still had to think and analyze and conjecture. I couldn't just be. And then I did just let myself go. Since then, I've just kind of been floating around. I've had the nicest, calmest, most serene feelings I've ever had.

For once, I just let myself be. I didn't make it a reward or a condition or make its happening depend on other things (like losing weight or something else) happening first. I just let it (no made it) happen to me. And felt it was the best thing I'd ever done.

So am I scared of this—this just being—instead of contriving or manipulating? I like it the other way, I want it the other way, but on days like today I feel like I'm screwing it up, and don't really understand why.

JANUARY 20

I started writing something, and I ripped it up. It started to take on a depressing tone, but that's not how I feel. Today (and that's all that matters) I feel good. There are no conscious reasons for it. What a relief, I don't have to *make* myself feel okay anymore.

My eyes are open wider. My mind is open wider. I have hope again. I'm moving in a positive direction as opposed to a negative one. Not being perfect. Just being.

I think when I started decaying is when I stopped everything else. I'll feel better if I exercise, go to work, go to classes, instead of not going because I'm not "up to it." I always get surprised and feel better when I *do,* when I live. I don't want to retreat into a shell and hide. Sometimes I feel that way, but it's not what I really want.

Things don't have to be *either* wonderful *or* awful anymore. There is an in between. I know because I'm in it right now, and it's so much easier than the *burden* of each extreme.

JANUARY 26

Dear Lisa,

I received your letter just the other day. To tell the truth, I was somewhat taken aback by it. Both by what you wrote and the way you wrote it. I feel that you must have changed a bit since we last spoke, and the change suits you well. Clearly, your life must be taking *definite* shape because your writing reflects a new confidence and assertiveness that I didn't recognize before.

More than that, your remarks about my letter were probably quite just. I wish I could read it again to see if I really did say things the way you said I did. You wield an accurate pen, but I won't turn this card into a rebuttal. What I really want to do is wish you a *Happy Birthday,* and say that I'm glad that you, like I also said, want to get together. I hope that we will do so very soon. I sense that there is still much we have to say and learn from one another. The best way to do that is face to face.

Love,
Perry

FEBRUARY 1

Dear Perry,

What a nice card you sent me. I'm glad you want to get together. I had an idea about that. What about the end of February? It could mark the second anniversary of our first date. (Remember that?)

I'm glad you didn't use your card as a rebuttal. I had thought of that word, "rebuttal," before, while writing my letter. I thought, God, what is this, a debate or an argumentative essay? When I realized that's what it was turning into, I stopped because that's not what I had intended. You're right, if my letter seemed strong, I guess it does reflect a strength or assertiveness that's developed in me and enables me to stand up for myself.

You know, to be honest (which is what we said we'd be, right?) even though I was the one who said we shouldn't fool ourselves, I think we have been a little. I'm not sure how to put it, or what, in fact, it really is, but, whereas I can say to you, "Yes, let's be friends" (and I really want that to happen), I can't act that way. For instance, if I were dealing with another friend now who is ten minutes away, I'd call to make plans. Somehow that's not an easy thing to do in this situation. This is more complicated (feelings-wise), but like you said, I'm sure it will be worth it.

I used to feel as if I had no basis or foundation to pull from—like a person fumbling around in the dark. I don't feel that way anymore. And I have to tell you it's one of the most freeing experiences I have had. Maybe you don't feel that way anymore either (or maybe I'm presuming too much to think that you ever felt that way, but I don't think so, and that happened to be one of the things I liked about you at the time).

Even if you do still feel that way, that's okay. People are entitled to be on different timetables or in different places. You know, that's so easy to see now, that we were never "in the same place at the same time." If we were, I (we, probably) didn't know it. You know, I had you married before we even went out on a date. Did I ever tell you that I thought I wanted to marry you in eighth grade when we met in speech and debate class?! I thought, "I've found him." Tell me, who in eighth grade thinks these things? Then in ninth and tenth grade, before we finally got together our senior year, I had other crushes as well as boys who proclaimed their love for me, but never another situation where I thought like that.

Oh, there's other newer stuff I want to tell you. I think I understand some of the ways you acted in relation to me that I never did before. You see, my friend, I think we're more alike than it might appear because put in a situation similar to yours I acted remarkably similarly. I was pursued by someone who was "so sure," "really sure" I was the *one*. Well, I liked him, a lot, but this quick seriousness petrified me. I wouldn't commit under any circumstances. I would make no commitments, take no risks. I can't think of them now, but I actually said things that you had said.

You know what it was, though, *fear* and way too much control over myself. Well, it's funny what's happened, I let down my guard, and let myself be natural. I'm not scared anymore, and I feel I've gained more real control (not the artificial control I had before).

I'm not trying to paint this as your picture. But I do think that what I used to think of as an incredible high moral attitude and righteousness on your part was probably partly fear (for lack of a better word). An uppity moral attitude and righteousness are, in my opinion, questionable as to whether they're assets or liabilities. Fear, on the other hand, is a perfectly human, endearing emotion.

Maybe through your newer relationship you've discovered some of the same things that I have. But I have to (or want to) mention a recent observation. Not to go into rebuttal, but at the end of your letter, you mentioned the girl you've been seeing, you said you were doing it so as not to be hypocritical about being honest and upfront (or perhaps, about leading me on?). Well, I didn't think about it until well after I sent my letter, but I wrote about David (my new person) because it was a big, nice, exciting thing that had happened to me. I started thinking that you didn't mention *at all* how you (or if you) felt about this girl. (Probably because you didn't think it appropriate, or most likely any of my business.) But anyway, I thought it was interesting that she was only brought up in relation to you and me. You said you were telling me so as not to "deceive" me. That's not something you tell to a friend. It's something you tell to a girlfriend. You're not deceiving a friend if you don't tell them about a girlfriend because the friend has no *vested* interest.

I hope you're not upset with my honesty. But I do live differently now. When I get confused, upset, or faced with misconceptions, I just don't bury it. I try and clear it up in my mind. Believe me (you may already know) it makes any important relationship better.

Believe it or not, this started out to be a very short note. You're right, we probably do still have a lot to tell each other. But face to face?! I'm sure after all of this time, it'll be interesting, s-c-a-r-y, and very worthwhile.

I'm looking forward to hearing from you.

Love,
Lisa

(I decided it wasn't important enough anymore to send.)

FEBRUARY 14

See Dick. Dick wants you to be *Happy* on Valentine's Day! Happy! Happy! See Jane. Jane wants you to have *fun* on Valentine's Day! Fun! Fun! See Spot. Spot wants to jump in your lap and nibble your ears. Arf. Arf. As for me, I think Spot has the right idea! You are the sexiest devil I ever knew. I love you very much.

All my love,
David

* * * * *

When I'm calling you, you make my heart SING! Happy Valentine's Day.

Love,
David

* * * * *

Happy Valentine's Day . . . to someone who really knocks me out!

Love,
David

* * * * *

I'm a creature of habit! I think of you every five seconds!

Love,
David

FEBRUARY 22

And they said it wouldn't last! Happy six-month anniversary.

Love,
David

* * * * *

Congratulations. As always a brilliant performance. Six months and *All*-ways.

Love,
David

* * * * *

Lisa,

These have been the best six months of my life. All because of you. I love you very much.

> Love,
> *David*

You get such a high because it's *you!* All you have. What else is there? What else is the point?

On Just Moving Home for Summer

Yesterday, Dad and I took my car in to be fixed. We went out to breakfast. We played tennis. We drove to the store together. Today, we played tennis again. Five sentences. Just five sentences. But, oh, what they imply.

We talked. Not just school. Not just money. In fact, rarely school, barely money. We actually had conversations that were a lot closer to interpersonal discussions. Damn close, in fact.

What's gone is the paranoia, the fear of judgment, the certainty of not measuring up. Or rather, the terror of appearing to measure up, but, in reality, not holding a candle to the image, the façade.

We're not all of a sudden soul mates, buddies, pals. But, then again there is that glimmer that says we two may be the most alike of us all.

In other words, all these years we've been fooled, or fools. Lisa looks like Mom. Lisa is like Mom. Lisa is Mom. My brother looks like Dad. But, then again, not as much as Lisa looks like Mom. And, besides, my brother has always been himself, not a reflection, not a puddle.

Maybe looks are deceiving. I may look like Mom, but I'm beginning to see I'm a combination of both parents. I'm not like Mom. I'm not like Dad. I'm the indescribable essence that is both of them. Thus, I am unique.

Now that I have come to accept my uniqueness without malice, as well as without exaggerated awe and glorification, I have reached a soothing, calming balance. Needless to say then, it is no longer the chemicals or calories in food that soothe and calm me.

Being at peace like this has unlocked a little door somewhere on my body through which I have floated. For once, being able to get outside of myself. I slipped out, however, for more than some air and a little sightseeing. I broke out to join forces with my alter ego, my soul mate, my love. David is the acceptance, the support, and the true know-you-inside-and-out-and-still-want-you-no-matter-what love that I never allowed myself to believe conceivable in the past.

That past, though, is becoming less and less of a burden to haul around. It lives on in the pages of this journal. It lives on, too, in a little corner of my mind. There's no rent control, though, in that particular corner. The rates for staying on keep getting higher and higher. Few of those old-timers can afford to pay, so they're packing up and moving out, leaving room for newer, more amiable tenants.

MAY 24

Yesterday, I saw a mother and son crossing the street. There was some traffic. Not a lot, but some. The mother went first, not even watching the kid, let alone holding his hand. Indifferent. Uncaring. Self-absorbed. Nevertheless, it was the only kid I've ever seen look for himself while crossing the street.

MAY 27

My last "booger" just fell out. You know, those booger scabs that had been filling, almost completely, my nostrils for months and months. I couldn't resist picking them out knowing there would again be blood, there would again be a scab. Over and over again the process, the cycle, was repeated. And now, finally, since I waited, hadn't thought about it for days and days, the last of the booger scabs has left. Naturally. Without my force. Just naturally.

JUNE 3

No matter what happens in my life, something must stay constant, a feeling of self-validation, the feeling of satisfaction with self. No matter what, this must *be*.

I've got to take care of myself. If I don't, who will? David will. My mom and dad will. That's the point, if I don't take over, keep charge, they will. And, unfortunately, they couldn't do half as good a job as I could.

JUNE 7

Oh, how things change. Everything in my life has changed, and amazingly I have not. I no longer change my personality to fit my mood. I don't feel like I'm a compound of different people anymore. I am just one person. I live. I breathe. I cope. I don't retreat. I don't escape. I don't muzzle myself.

JUNE 22

I did that thing, that special thing regarding professional writing, that I wanted to do while I was young, younger than would be expected of me. (Maybe it'll go, maybe it won't, but I still did it.)

JUNE 25

I've got a life.

Amazement. Wonder. Splendor. I've got a life. Not just the shell, but the core.

JULY 6

If I could be thin, I could have a whole new life. The only trouble is that I don't want a whole new life anymore.

JULY 8

I want to be like I was even though I didn't like it when I was there.

Someday, will I yearn to be as I am now, even though now, while I'm here, I don't like my weight either?

JULY 8

You plan a whole life, but you can't even picture six years of waiting. That's scary.

You thought, "I'm thinking marriage too soon." I could wait until I'm twenty-eight. No, then David would be thirty-one. Too old. Me twenty-seven. Him thirty. Hey, let's give the guy a break and shoot for under thirty. Me twenty-six. Him twenty-nine. Good.

We can date each other and others, fool around with each other and others for the time being. Then we could move in together one year after I get out of college. Twenty-three and a half. And live together for two and a half years. Marriage at twenty-six. Gives both of us enough time to be (really) sure. And the folks enough time to save up for the mega-wedding.

Lesson 281:
Don't discuss with your mother possibilities of future sex with as-of-now-unknown people. Even if you're indirect, she'll catch on.

Second Thought (Hot Flash via phone conversation):
You can't be all too sure about waiting when your heart feels like it's melting into a warm, soft mush and you just want to lie down and be hugged *by him*.

JULY 10

It would be so much less risky to playact with David. Make me so much less vulnerable to playact it "cool." It's so much more of a relief, though, not to have to.

JULY 13

I haven't been thin for a year and three months. And it hurts. It hurts.
Current Weight: 137.

JULY 13

It really shocked me the other day at work at the TV studio to see that hit singer in shorts and think she has the greatest body and know mine could never be that fantastic. Then I realized that I had looked the same way in shorts once. After all, I'd worn a size three. I guess I'd forgotten or pushed it outside of my mind.

JULY 15

I'm not going to fall back into the isolation. I'm not going to cut myself off from My World. I'm not going to crawl back into my yellow wallpapered shell with the rose-colored trim. God, I'm getting beckoned again, though.

But do I have to go? Succumb? Retreat? No, No, No. No, No, No, No. In fact, No Way.

I can keep going, keep moving, keep the circulation going. I can listen to the directions from the cynic in me with one ear so that I can move with both feet in the opposite direction!

JULY 16

I know I've changed because I can get out of a "down" without going deeper. Before, when I'd start feeling depressed, that's what it was, a start of a who knows how long depression. Days? Weeks? Months? Periods of feeling bad that directly followed periods of feeling good. I can, and often did, look back on my life and vividly remember it in blocks of happy months or blocks of despairing months. No balance. No in-between. Just a seesaw existence.

But now there's no more seesaw. I no longer spend all of my energy swinging up and down on a board that's going nowhere. I move. I may be unhappy, but I don't wallow and stagnate. It's not that I move because I tell, prod, or force myself to, either. I don't need any telling, prodding, or forcing. It just happens. This week, for example, I felt caught in a rut. Everything—David, job, family, education—fell flaw side up. However, maybe because I'm not cluttered and paralyzed with those subconscious demons anymore, my mind and body now actually have a natural, uninhibited response to such a situation–action. I worked out a whole course of study at school involving my first choice, marketable double major (journalism and women's studies). All of a sudden, my education seems worthwhile. I went to the TV newsroom at the studio where I work (the focus that pulled me in there off the street in the first place three years ago!) asking about weekend internships and jobs. All of a sudden, since there won't be anything available for months, my TV page job there seems worth holding onto. I initiated talks, discussions, fights with David. All of a sudden, my precious gem of a David seems worth insuring. When this mood nosedive started, I thought, "Oh, no, could I fall into that pit again?" My question has been more than answered.

JULY 17

Another thing that helped me realize how unconstructive this and possible future down moods are was my discussion with Anita Siegman, now in private practice for eating disorders, not at USC any longer.

I looked her up because I felt I still might need someone to talk to, and I didn't want to go back to Francine and have her think I was sliding backwards.

I asked her, "Will I ever be normal? Will I ever be like people who never worry about what they eat and stay trim?"

This had begun to worry me. Here I am, so much better than when I started out at the beginning of college, but it hit me that, although my attitudes are very different, I still eat "good stuff" in private. Even though I feel pretty good at a weight higher than I would have accepted before, and even though I don't really binge anymore, I still think I use food sometimes.

"Will I ever be normal?"

Anita brought up a good point. She said I'm not sick. There is nothing wrong with me. Unfortunately, she said, we live in a society where this kind of concern for weight and body is virtually "normal." She said, "You know, you've lived this way for years. You can't just necessarily expect it to go away completely in a year or two."

Thinking about it this way has made me feel better.

SEPTEMBER 16

So, should I say I am living with David? Not officially. No name on the mailbox or answering machine (he says he doesn't want that yet). Not paying much at all. But I am here.

It really started when Dad said, "So, will you be home tonight?" For weeks, I had been running past the kitchen when no one was looking with an overnight bag, then coming back in empty-handed and saying goodnight. Later, I would call and say I was too tired to drive home, etc.

I was surprised at the question. He said, "Come on, you're an adult now, and David's working and out of school. We trust your judgment. We know it's a different world now."

So, then, gradually I started moving stuff in, and now I have half the clos-

```
                        BBW
                        BIG
                     Beautiful
                       WOMAN
         Magazine Fashions for the Large-Size Woman

     Lisa Messinger
     7089 Cardinal Drive
     Encino, CA

     Dear Lisa,
          Thank you for sending us your manuscript, "I was a Teenage
     Fresca Freak." We are always happy to receive and review
     articles. We love your article, want to publish it and want
     you to contact us about contributing more writing to the
     magazine.
          BBW Magazine provides a national forum in which to expose
     writing talent. Many of our contributors have found being
     published in a national magazine to be a solid stepping stone
     into acquiring further freelance experience.
          Please sign and return the enclosed release form.
          Again, we appreciate your interest in BBW!
```

et. The nights I'd come back home he'd call and we'd talk, and we couldn't stand being apart. It was the most magnetic feeling I've felt for someone, drawn.

I have my own TV page friends, friends from USC, and my old friends, but I study a lot. He has so many friends and parties and I don't always want to go. This is causing some rift. He wants me to go with him, says he needs me for his entertainment law career. But I have homework, and I don't like going. I feel so, as of yet, unaccomplished. I'm a junior in college, a little page, and these people are *big* in the entertainment field.

David says, you should be more confident, more sure of how special you are, and that these people want to hear what you have to say. "Don't worry," he says, "I'll teach you to work a room."

I don't know. I know I'm drawn to David. And now, I'm a ninety percent of the time part of his apartment, the apartment I have always loved so much, and felt so at home at.

DECEMBER 15

"A Gender History" Introduction (USC, Women's Studies 210)

I dared to believe that I was different. I dared to believe that the world had changed. Now there is an emptiness inside of me, because I see that nothing has changed and that I could become another obliging victim. I had dared to believe that I would be able to pursue a career to its utmost, cataclysmic limits and have a passionate, thriving, close marriage as well.

My boyfriend, however, the man I want to marry, a man who believes in me and all of my possibilities as well as believing in the rights of women, has told me that he doesn't see how this blend is possible. It's because of *my* chosen profession. It's because I'm going to be a broadcast journalist. He sees no way I could rise near the top (where I would like to be and he feels I should be) without spending "some time" on the East Coast. His chosen career, entertainment law, necessitates staying on the West Coast, and therein lies the rub.

We could work it out, I said. We could have a bicoastal marriage, a house in California and an apartment in New York and commute on weekends, I said. That's not my idea of a marriage, he said. I want to have you near me, not 3,000 miles away, he said.

I guess I thought that if you were going to be with someone for the next fifty years, a few years of stolen weekends and leading exciting, thriving lives wouldn't be out of the question. I guess I thought that finding the right person was more important than finding someone whose schedule was compatible to yours, enabling them to be "near" you at all times. I guess I thought love was enough to work it out. I guess I was wrong.

First, I felt cheated because I am only twenty, and I'm already seeing possible limitations to a full and satisfying life. I'm already seeing that women still, to one degree or another, are asked to lead an "either/or" existence. Later, I just started to feel crazy for even considering that such an alternative lifestyle was even possible or reasonable. Anyone I mentioned it to seemed to think it wasn't. Living away from your mate is no way to have a marriage. You're only asking for problems, especially in the fidelity department, they all said. So, now I feel frustrated, crazy, selfish, and right all at the same time, a blend of feelings with which I am sure countless women, present and past, have struggled.

DECEMBER 17

I care about quality. I don't want my career to rest on ratings, a pretty smile, or the right time slot. That's not why I'm going into broadcast journalism. I'm studying broadcast journalism and women's studies at USC so that I can make poignant, pressing, probing documentaries about important social issues.

I have chosen documentaries because I want my career to be more than a three-minute segment on the six o'clock news. I have more than that to say. I am a public speaker and a writer, a writer who wants to reveal, enlighten, and amuse.

I see documentary making as one of my ultimate career goals. Your project sounds fascinating, the precise subject matter in which I am interested. I would love to start my career journey as a member of your team!

[Got the job for a documentary company that went on to later produce some of the most successful serious reality shows of all time.]

JANUARY 11

Dear Ms. Abetta:

I have known since I was sixteen years old when I stepped into the CBS newsroom as a reporter's "shadow-for-a-day" that broadcast journalism was the life for me. That's the sole reason I chose to come to USC—since it was one of the few schools offering a degree in broadcast journalism. I know the field requires more than just classroom experience, though. That's why I have been trying to lay a solid working foundation as well. Although I am just turning twenty-one, I have already been working at a TV station in television production for two and a half years. At this point, I am very eager to move into the television newsroom. I think your newscast is done excellently, and that you have the best local news/talk show in Los Angeles. I would very much like to be associated with your station in the news intern position that is available.

I have included a copy of my resumé.

JANUARY 25

Laura Abetta
TV News Assignment Editor

Dear Ms. Abetta:

I really enjoyed meeting you the other day. Thank you for offering me the news internship, especially since it didn't fit in with the UCLA intern's schedule. Believe it or not, however, since I spoke with you, I interviewed and was chosen for a part-time job at the TV station where I've been working for two and a half years. I will be the programming assistant in the programming department. I will answer all viewer concerns and assist the program director and the two program managers, and I am looking forward to it to get even more experience before I move into a job in their TV newsroom.

Thanks again for the offer, but I think I will stick with my current TV studio for the time being.

Sincerely,
Lisa Messinger

JANUARY 26

What to do? Have I imagined this? What happened to the sweet man I fell in love with who was *madly* in love with me and would do anything for me?

Nothing I do seems to be right. He criticizes almost everything I do. Maybe I am doing everything wrong. That's how he makes me feel. I have to come out of my shell or I'll lose him, and our life, the life that "will never be boring." If he leaves me alone, I'll be boring. Why did he change? Or was he always like this and acted that way to get me hooked?

I love David very much and I want to make him happy. I know that I have certain personality deficiencies and parts that aren't developed yet, but he can help me. I know he can.

And he's been my one confidante, the one person who knows everything in the world about me, all my problems past and present. And he's let me share his fun life. I think I probably should make some or most of the changes he says I should. I'll try.

I just don't think I can party all the time, or even a half, or a quarter, or an eighth of the time. I'll just try and grin and bear it and be more open to it.

JANUARY 31

Dear Mr. Sorrell,

This is something I wanted to tell you when you were visiting from Chicago. In fact, I wanted to tell you before I even met you. I wanted to say thank you. Thank you because you have created the most wonderful combination of a person I could think of in David. I knew as I got to know him that he had to have some remarkable parents to have grown into the special person that is him. Somewhere, somebody taught him and showed him what it is to be a loving, caring, giving, warm, sensitive, sweet, beautiful person. All along, I knew it had to be you. Just the way David talks about you—you can tell that he is very happy when anyone compares you. And after meeting you, I can see why.

I just wanted to say that I hope you are feeling better and thank you for creating a young man who is so easy to love.

Lisa

MARCH 14

No personality—wishy-washy—no opinions.
Unresponsive—insensitive.
Not friendly enough with people.
Don't *know how* to help him with his pain.

He can't tell me, I should just know he's in pain, just like he knows for me without words.

Put my pain on him, he can't be my psychoanalyst anymore, I talk too much about my problems—what about his?

I won't wear a bathing suit.

I'm *dragging him down* like dead weight—he has to drag me to things.

I'll never do anything wrong. We have different priorities. Our values are different. Mine: scholarship, guilt. His: fun, parties.

After eighteen months, not enough in common, like sports or politics.

No stimulation.

No stimulating discussions for months.

No emotional stimulation.

I don't have it in me to change.

He's been giving—doesn't feel he's gotten anywhere as much back. Can't give anymore.

He loves me. Will feel empty without me.

There's no future for us. He can't marry me, seeing the way I am.

Doesn't have patience to wait to see if I can change anymore.

I wrote this all down so I don't just let go of it, go on and do nothing about it. With or without him, I'm going to do something.

MARCH 15

1) Go see school counselor regarding my social problems.
   (She said I don't seem to have any problems.)
2) Join Sally's Figuretique ($149 for two years)
   I am going to lose ten pounds so I can feel comfortable wearing a bathing suit this summer.
3) Sit and wait at David's.
4) Tell him about 1 & 2. I am going to change.

MARCH 16

A.M.

Sit and wait at David's all day, but he doesn't come home.

P.M.

Tell him again he's wrong—I have it in me to change—that he's making this decision because his father is very ill and he's upset.

He said that's not the reason. We're just not right for each other, but maybe we can just cool it a while, not go out as exclusively. We'll call for dates, etc. That's when I knew I got him back.

MAY 8

Well, he died. His heart battered him and broke him down, and then just refused to tick. They gave each other a fight until the end. David's father is dead, and there's nothing I can do about it. No way I can help him with his pain. Because he will not let me. He will barely speak. He sleeps and sleeps and sleeps. When he's awake, he wants to try and have fun and forget.

I can't forget. I cannot sleep it off. I can't forget his problems and I can't forget mine. What about the idiot who bashed into my car? What about the doctor who was treating me for my ankle after the car accident and decided he'd heard so much about me from my aunt that he felt he knew me? What difference did it make that he was forty-five and married? No twenty-three-year-old guy could appreciate me, the brilliance behind my eyes, he said.

He said it after the molestation, though. When I think I'm getting examined and I'm really getting felt up (and then kissed) by a sick doctor with a waiting room full of googly-eyed patients, I call that molest. David calls it too trivial to think about. After all, his problem is much worse, but then he won't talk about that.

JULY 1

Moment upon moment, I walk on eggshells.

I have it down to a science now.

Test question 1: "Will you go to the football game (that you hate) with us?"

"Why, yes, Sir. Of course, Sir."

There is no chance to say no now. Why rock the boat? If I say "No" now to anything, I don't know what'll happen.

I have learned to play the game. Finally. So well, in fact, he doesn't know I'm playing. He thinks this is really me now. I like to party now. I like to go out all the time. Hup. Hup. Keep moving. Who'd ever want to be alone?

He thinks this is really me. And now if I step out of character, he'll know the truth. And I'll have blown everything I've worked for.

AUGUST 20

Happy Birthday, David.

"Nothing yields more pleasure and content to the soul than when it finds that which it may love fervently, for to love and live beloved is the soul's paradise."

—WILLIAM BRADFORD, 1630

I hope you like the cashmere sweater, it'll make you only that much more softer to hug.

Love,
Lisa

SEPTEMBER 15

2:17 A.M.

If you love someone, let them go, if it was meant to be, they'll fly back to you.
David Sorrell-
Lisa Messinger

I don't feel the same need to hold on right now. I feel the only way it will work is if he *really* wants me. And I don't feel that I can "make" that happen. I don't feel, even, that if he doesn't feel it that I'm any less (of a person). Oddly enough, I'm left with the impression that he thinks more of me than I thought he did. So, I feel ahead. I have my own good impression of myself as well as his.

I feel that I have no idea what might happen, but I do not now feel devastated or totally depleted. I feel like there's a lot in me. Not near enough, though, to change David. If he changes, *he* changes. I don't change him, and I don't change me to change him. That, of course, is what I was doing before. Now I'm calmer (?) because I know it can't be done.

I believe I will be okay regardless of what becomes.

LATER: This is good, whether for a period or forever, because it pushes, if not forces, me to decide what I really want to do with my life.

Thank God I am not in a position where I feel I should not be, someplace I went because of David. Thank God, even though that played heavily and I might be, probably would be, in a different place without him, thank God at this point I am at a place that feels right to me.

I actually, whether falsely or not, feel strong. Actually strong? Now that he's made the final break. I don't feel like I did the last time, which, although I won't go into it, was a disaster. Hell on tears. Last time my initial reaction was to try and change myself to fit his mold. Now, somehow, I have gotten far from there. (I just pictured myself laughing tomorrow.) Not thinking about this every minute. Getting on. Without a cookie-cut future. Perhaps to write again.

Of course, I saw this, although not obvious. Turning off sad soap operas—dealing with death of the loved one—I cried and couldn't watch. I never cry over soap and death. Reaching out to David's friends, trying to pull him in (on the reel, like a fish) through them.

I need time to myself, or I'll be smothered. In a not-right situation, I'll never know. It was, of course, too early or too late, or somewhere in the middle, but not the right time. I tear as I say, why don't we believe the people who say, timing is everything.

12. Real Life
21 TO 22 YEARS OLD

I'm so glad I moved back to this university-owned beautiful apartment and lucked out and got such nice, wonderful roommates but . . .

Most good writing comes out of pain. Why is it that today I feel like crying? Not yesterday or the day before, but today. Today I could have just as easily have stayed in bed. Indeed, lay on the bed most of the day. Soap opera. Soap opera. Shed a soapy tear. TV prompts it. Real life put it there ready to spring from the aqueduct.

As I glance at the "I" that is written, I feel guilt. What's the use of picking it all apart? Why, why be so concentrated on self? I haven't been for a long time, and it's been good. Yea, baby, life's been good to me. That's something you don't like to give up. It's hard to understand why you have to.

I never really have put David on paper very much. Two years of my life lived, but not on paper. That's what I did, I lived. Raw and real, not self-conscious or hung up, but action, motion, lust, and love *in the flesh*. Part of me wants to say I love David so much and part and part and part—I don't know. Here I am all by my lonesome, la, la, la.

Here I am a normal person. With normal lusts and desires. I'm a fucking normal person, and I feel connected with the world at large. I can relate and understand and plug into those and that around me. I am part of the human condition and I feel it.

I want to have sex. It's that plain and simple. Now that I have floated to this spot that does not include dwelling on David, I want others. Not just one, but several. Just for the physical. I want a lover. Someone with whom I can be physical (often) and yet remain myself—some distance—to be just me. Not a part of a bigger something. Only me, with a lover. A young stud, attentive but not smothering. And great in bed and to me. Later a real love and lover. Right now, I could truly get into some serious fucking.

(A part of me says I'm writing this way to shock compared to last writings years ago. Part says, "Fuck, that's who I am now.")

DECEMBER 13

You realize the significance of the date, of course. I did, when I wrote it. And before, thinking what I was doing two years ago, to date.

Fucking, that's what. Losing it for the first time. Coming the first time and thinking, WOW, I thought nobody did that the first time. Wow, what a great sex life I'm going to have. Ah, the grand expectation.

Not that it wasn't fulfilled. Just nowhere near wholly. Mainly, in the end, I had a very good sex life because of myself. I learned how to *really* do it well and was totally at ease with this man and he was very at ease with me being the one to really go at it.

Now, re-evaluation is at mind. I haven't changed quite as much as I might have thought. When it seemed that push was going to come to shove, I thought long and quite hard about what I really wanted to do. My body, very definitely, craved the touch in every cavern and space. Every cavern and space wanted to be filled, longed for it. But then, from somewhere inside, all of those parental adolescent warnings started talking, "What will you feel about it tomorrow? Don't you want it to be with someone special?" Yes, yes, yes. I realized that the same things mattered to me as had before. Yearnings, yes. Horniness, hell, yes. But with anybody, anything male? No, thank you. I'm exaggerating a bit, of course, after all, since he's an acquaintance of David's and I've already known him for more than a year and he was always extremely sweet to me, not to mention extremely cute.

I'm still not jumping for joy. But I am okay. Everything and nothing is up for grabs. The same old things are still the same old things, and yet everything is different. I realize the good in my own personal, very own, life. And I still have, somehow intact, every hope for the future.

DECEMBER 18

The Lisa takes a lover. A lover. A lover. There are other ways to be happy that somehow come from within and through other people. Add one lover and blend well.

So the Lisa took a lover. A lover. A lover. Smoldering fires must eventually be extinguished or fed. Or both.

Nourishing myself is what I'm doing. I can see it at work. I am being nourished by the friendship and experience of the older (somewhat) women. Being nourished at home by the young spirit of the college co-eds I call wondrous to be around. Nourished by my family, my friends. For all the nourishing I did, only to end up malnourished and shockingly dehydrated.

Sperm, enter me and nourish me. Nourish me. Nourish and flourish I will.

I am flourishing as an individual. And within that flourishing, I can be nourished and cherished by those who surround me.

I'm (I am) glad.

DECEMBER 20

You know something, I just realized I still weigh 140 pounds. And around Thanksgiving I weighed around 143. And you know what, weight doesn't even matter to me anymore. I just eat what I want, when I want, and that's it. I don't binge, ever. That is simply not a response anymore. I don't force myself not to, it just would be an unnatural action for me now. I also don't use food at all, because I know I can have whatever I want whenever I want it in front of whomever I want to.

JANUARY 8

You're on your own, kid. That's what crossed my mind in the bathroom. Funny, what crosses the mind in the bathroom. That was the first time I've really felt that way.

Something else that crossed my mind today. I am happy, and effortlessly so. I just happened to realize how happy I am and have been. It's just this thing I've been living in without really thinking about it.

And I realized that all of the things that made me realize I was happy had solely to do with me, stemmed just from me. The people who are helping make my life full now are my people. They don't belong to someone else and merely populate my life. They're my friends, my roommates, my family, my dates. My workmates. Wow, they really are all my people. What I was missing out on before! Taking seconds on someone else's picks.

My job (career) decisions. Actually decisions. My advances toward that special one of the opposite sex who had always expressed his desire for me. And, of course, I didn't just haphazardly "take a lover," as I excitedly wrote about him on December 18. I had wanted him for a year and he had made me feel special that hard year, even though he had a different attractive date every night, with his constantly saying, "I know you're David's girlfriend, but all I want is a girlfriend like you." Our relationship—even though I know we are so different and will inevitably go our own ways soon—has been eye opening.

Ups and downs, downs and ups, yes. But, mostly, a calm, nice up. Everything, me, is just damn okay.

JANUARY 15

An interesting thought crossed my mind. I am proud of myself in a different way than before, in a way that says, I'm glad I made my life full and that I'm living and enjoying it.

Working in the television newsroom for the first time at the TV studio where I've worked for the last three years with just that goal in mind seems to be something to record for posterity. There will, of course, never be first time again. I'm in, and that's about all there is to it. The news manager said after my final interview that I had more chutzpah than anyone he'd met. He said he thought, "That girl has chutzpah, I'm going to find something for her."

David calls and the complications begin. Because no matter how wrong everyone now believes he is for you—you, of course, cared about him.

JANUARY 29

I can't think of what to write
because everything is just so okay.
I feel calm. I feel content.
I feel happy.
There's no man, no pinpoint
reason for this feeling of good.
There's a life, a lifestyle, being
lived by a fully functioning individual.
I can take care of myself.
What more could I ask for?
Now I can truly feel that no matter
what I have or don't have, I truly have
all I need, all I'll ever need.

FEBRUARY 20

Hey there, ho there, hi there. Footloose and fancy-free and feeling fine. Feeling like what it's like to really feel again. Maybe for a night, but maybe not, and that's the thrill of it.

Feeling I've seen a bit and picked, Josh, one gem-type from the pool. Not the pool of life—but the pool of the months. Making him the most interesting of the interesting to bounce by.

Oh, la la. What bouncing this has had me doing.
It must be something when your life seemed the farthest thing from lonely, and then this person bounces in and it seems that if they're gone and not there you'll be a little lonely for them.

How come I didn't feel the least bit lonely 'til I met him and he's not here every minute?

What the hell has happened? One date and the girl's gone around the bend.

Dear Josh,

Unfortunately, the episode titled "Things That Go Creep In the Night" of the one-hour drama that you appeared in isn't creeping at the moment. Our TV station does show the program in reruns, but we've had print problems with it, and have not been able to air it as of yet. We probably won't be able to schedule it until May.

Since you were the guest star on that episode, I'm sorry we couldn't have given you better news. I'd like to be able to get a dub for you, but I checked into it, and, unfortunately, I can't.

The only reason you get such special treatment, if you want to call it that, is because of your New York accent. I've been talking on these phones for almost a year now (I go to USC, write for a magazine, and work in the TV station's newsroom, too), and, after our long conversation, you have to rank with the most interesting people with whom I've spoken.

Listen, I'm a nice Jewish girl, and I hope everything works out for you. Call if we can help you with anything else, or if you want to check on the status of the show, or if you want to brighten up a day otherwise filled with nowhere near as interesting viewer calls.

Good luck,

Lisa Messinger

Lisa Messinger
Programming Assistant

FEBRUARY 24

Even other women tell women to sit around and wait for a man to confirm their validity and desirability. Did he call yet? Why should he have to call?

If I know there's something to be interested in here, and every cell is telling me to do something about it—that I will feel good if I do: validated, confirmed, alive, vital, in control of my future—why shouldn't I?

I knew that I'd feel better if *I* did something rather than if I waited and he

From the Concerned TV Programming Staff:

Questionnaire for Mr. Josh Levine upon the Occasion of His Going Out for the First Time with Ms. Lisa Messinger, Lovely Young Thing Who Must Not Be Abused.

1. How old are you, Mr. Levine?
   - A. 20 years
   - B. 25 years
   - C. over 30
   - D. elderly

2. Why don't you have a car, Mr. Levine?
   - A. Can't afford it
   - B. Couldn't pass the test
   - C. I like to sponge off friends
   - D. New Yorkers don't like cars

3. What type of TV shows have you appeared on?
   - A. Comedy sitcom
   - B. Late-night nudes
   - C. Dating game show

4. How do you think of Ms. Messinger? You think she is . . .
   - A. Wild, ready to be tamed
   - B. Innocent, like a lovely child
   - C. Sassy, with a gypsy fire
   - D. Un Schickte Fleish Mit Sve Egen
     (the Yiddish term for a boring piece of meat with two eyes)

5. As an actor, which of these things would you never do?
   - A. Appear nude
   - B. Appear clothed
   - C. Appear intelligent
   - D. Appear in front of an audience

6. You think of yourself as another . . .
   - A. Robin Williams
   - B. Tom Hanks
   - C. Mickey Mouse
   - D. Gumby
   - E. No one—I am unique

7. What is your most-prized possession?
   - A. My monogrammed underwear
   - B. My portrait portfolio
   - C. My letter from Lisa

8. If it comes to that, where will you and Lisa get married?
   - A. On a romantic stretch of Malibu beach
   - B. Married? You kidding?
   - C. Anywhere she wants
   - D. A tacky Las Vegas chapel

Thank you very much for your cooperation in this matter.

did something. After all, he had called for the first date. The point was my taking responsibility for getting something to happen that I wanted. Why should I leave my fate—a fate that I definitely have an interest in—in someone else's hands?

It's not as though I didn't have encouragement. It's not as if he didn't say he wanted to go out with me again. He did say it and gave me every indication it was true. So, why the hell sit around and wait, deciding that he was a rotten liar.

Why sully the real niceness of the evening by afterthoughts caused by the paranoid mind of a waiting, helpless woman?

I felt good today because of what I did, not because of what he said. I don't need a man to make me feel good about myself anymore. Since that feeling comes from me, I'm free to do anything I damn well please.

Catch up, everyone.

FEBRUARY 26

I weigh 130 pounds, and last night, Josh, a man (special!), was telling me what a great body I have. Huggable, kissable, delicious. This is not something I want to record for posterity, but, hey, thirteen pounds are gone and I don't feel like I really did a damn thing to lose them.

I'm a taster of life now. A participant. A liver.

I don't think I'm doing anything to prove anything to anyone. This is my life. I am young, and I want to live the way that seems most fulfilling to me. There are nowhere near as many no's as yes's these days.

I know who I am and what I want, and anything I do is not changing that. I'm proud of myself, not for blatantly external achievements, but for the way I'm grappling with these personal issues.

FEBRUARY 28

Everything is so good and right and fun. I have so many friends and people that I like. I'm in the TV newsroom learning, earning.

I love being with Josh, the funny, enchanting, especially cute actor from New York City who thinks I'm the best thing since sliced bread. But before him and during him and after him, I still have what I had, full happiness and basic contentment.

I think back to a few—three—years ago when I'd probably only be writing so cheerfully because of my body realignment. Not now. My God, I didn't even try to lose weight. It's just that going to school in the morning, working four hours in the TV station programming department in the afternoon, and working three nights a week in the TV newsroom left only time to eat for energy. My God, I didn't even *realize* until I stopped walking to school for winter break that

that's what had firmed up my legs and hips, kept me from gaining weight, and made me feel generally *good*. Believe it or not, this weight did just fall off, and it had nothing to do with the main focus of my life.

Of course, there must be some way things could be better, and things could certainly be worse, but I wouldn't trade places with anyone at all.

MARCH 20

David, I have a new lover now. Josh relishes my presence, my body. He tells me to hear him, that he is *making love* to me, nothing less. How can my eyes, brows, teeth, and body, which he loves, be so pretty? He whispered that in my ear.

I think I took this thirty-year-old man by surprise ("Too young, too cute. No, sorry, an emerging woman, the best I ever had").

Who knows how long? Who cares? That's not the point. We're the point. We connect. We fit. We make love, no matter how different we are.

I feel totally free and myself. Not afraid or concerned with tomorrow much. Too occupied with tonight.

Give him to me, and let me make love to him, and then let me go my way alone tomorrow.

All my fortunes came true.

MARCH 21

How can I explain how I feel? It's all happened. It's all here, and it's all me and now. I like everything and everything likes me.

Lick that ice cream cone, not because it's going to melt, but because it tastes *so* good.

I did it. I'm happy. I have more people around me now. So many more people I need, but truly dependent on no one.

I really like sex. So why shouldn't I have it? I really want life. So why shouldn't I live it? I really like Josh. So why shouldn't I see him?

Yawn. Go to sleep. Happy.

THERE'S A KILLER ON THE LOOSE . . . GRAB A NOOSE

BY LISA MESSINGER

Apparently, there's a killer on the loose in our neighborhood, and he may have been aided and abetted by members of the Greek fraternity/sorority community. If the story in the school newspaper is accurate, members of the Greek fraternity/sorority community helped a man who told them "he had just stabbed somebody and probably killed him."

Interestingly, this information was tucked away in the 27th paragraph of a 32-paragraph article. Perhaps the reporter, like those involved, didn't see this behavior as unacceptable. How, though, could it have been seen as anything but unacceptable?

Clearly, the fraternity and sorority members were in danger and should have acted accordingly. None of us would have expected them to endanger their lives and would have probably understood almost anything they had done to avoid being harmed. What they did do, however, seems highly questionable.

The article said a man who was covered with blood entered the fraternity house. He was confronted by approximately 25 fraternity and some sorority members. He told them he had been attacked by a gang of Mexicans. He said he had stabbed and probably killed someone, but as he was on parole, he didn't want the police to know about it.

While in the house, the article said, the man made a phone call and was given a pair of shorts by a fraternity member to replace his blood-stained sweatpants. Then, the article said, the fraternity members chased him from the house.

If these 25 young men were able to chase the man out of the house at that point, why was he able to make a phone call and given clothing beforehand? The article didn't mention anyone in the house calling the police. Couldn't at least one of the 25 have slipped away to make the call? Why, I think we should all ask, did they react as they did?

Perhaps it had something to do with the kind of reasoning that was behind this summation of the situation. "He seemed innocent," the fraternity member said. "He didn't seem like a ghetto person who wanted to kill anybody."

Well, according to the police and witnesses quoted in the article, apparently whatever man did want to kill somebody did so maliciously and violently, by not only shooting the man with a gun whose bullet grazed his head, but by going after the bleeding man and stabbing him to death.

Who, we should ask, put this fraternity member or any other in the position to judge and evaluate, or even contemplate, anyone's guilt or innocence? Now, no doubt due in part to that arrogant contemplation, there is a very good chance that a violent, wanted killer is roaming our streets or hiding out in our neighborhood.

Lisa Messinger is a senior in print journalism and the study of women and men in society.

MARCH 22

This will, of course, have to go down as the day I slept with two men within the scope of seven hours. Come home from one emergency room date with Josh and his bruised ribs from the movie scene he filmed today, and end up in bed with your supposed platonic friend and fellow student who tends to be madly in love with you. Of course, you were attracted to Christopher before you even met Josh and, on many an occasion, wondered just when and if he would kiss you. The game's the same I guess. Googly eyes and attraction. It's just that the stakes are higher now.

Well, I like Josh. And I like Christopher. For completely different reasons. And I guess that in part describes why I would have done this, and will probably continue doing it. At least with Christopher. I keep swinging back and forth between my different ideal sex partner types. Here I am starting up again with a healthy, perfectly built young man who knows nothing from clocks or time or nothing. All night long is how Lionel Richie put it in that old song, I believe.

Do I sound crass? I don't know? I gave my heart to David. It was loved and cherished and chewed up and spit out. Why should I be jumping to give it again? In the first place, I haven't met anyone yet who I'd really want to give it to right at this second. I like staying in control, and I don't see why I have to stay in control alone until someone who I will fall in love with comes along. Right now, high attraction in all areas seems enough. I like it. Why can't it be that simple? I knew with Christopher it might not be, that we are not in the same place, and he might want more. That stopped me for a while, but in the long run I know you can't be responsible for another person. You can care, but you can't create their experiences for them. What you have is what you have, and, hopefully, it will be good for both of you.

It's very exciting and ultimately healthy, I think, not to know exactly where you're going. I just know I'll get there, not how.

APRIL 1

Well, what can I say, except that I now know what great sex is. I know what it feels like to feel at one with another body. I know what it feels like not to have to move and yet to feel like you're floating on a cloud. There's no explaining why it's *so good* with this particular someone. It just is. It just feels so good. For so long.

I always thought that for it to be really good I had to move this way or that, really concentrate, participate, make it good for myself as much as they could have. Hey, hey, hey. Not so so so so. It feels so good.

Christopher is so inexperienced and yet so perfect.

He says he loves me. I am wonderful, beautiful, ambitious—a girl he thought was quiet and studied a lot. Now, he thinks I'm delectably wild, and all that's good—a girl he wants for hours upon end.

It's funny what one accidental stroke of the hand can lead to. It's all so delicious and warm and beautiful. I wonder if I can take a month and a half of it—until school gets out and he transfers—and all the rest of my months without him.

APRIL 4

Well, I finally made love on my own bed. Not in his apartment, or the other his apartment, or the extra bed in the other room. It's not a big deal, but it seemed the odds were against it. This has been my bed for over seven months and no one's shared it. Now I am a college girl in lust with a college boy, and even though that's not altogether true, it is. Sweet dreams.

APRIL 21

I feel elevated and airy. I know this is just a fling, and yet I know what utter delight is now. Just the physical. I've been mentally and mentally and mentally stimulated by rock managers and aspiring producer geniuses and entrepreneur-type architects.

Give me this bliss.

For another week and a half.

I can talk to my friends.

Only Christopher can make me fly right now.

APRIL 25

I haven't the energy after preparing eighteen units worth of final projects to think or walk or sleep, and yet I smile and am happy and am not annoyed or pained at the expulsion of my juice. Upstairs, I find and leave in Sarah, a friend among friends. What else could need filling? It's all there and within, waiting. Who could want more?

MAY 1

When you still remember the way David's robe felt, it hasn't been as long as you thought.

When you still remember the depth of the pockets, the little flicks of lint, it couldn't be that long.

When you remember getting out of his bed and putting on his robe and the way your body felt underneath, how could it have been that long?

It felt heavy like it was hanging on you, almost pulling you down.

Wondering if the newer one is wearing that robe makes you wonder just how long it's been.

And yet it's been quite a while, you think, when you catch a glimpse in your closet of the sexy black dress that jumped with Josh.

You didn't care then, and you don't care now, if she's in his robe because your sexy black dress and all your jeans and nice blouses have been wrinkled and smell like a wonderful actor who's about to return from a just-long-enough jaunt to the East Coast.

MAY 4

Well, he's transferring, and it's over, as I knew it would be. As, really, I want it to be. He's transferring out of my life.

Christopher is such a sweet boy. We have had a wonderful time. We both feel that way. This has been kind of dreamlike. Cocoonlike.

He says he loves me, is going to take the train up from San Diego and visit me a lot. He does not see how different we are. He does not know that it would not work.

He will have to see. I think he already does. It will do us no good, and there is no use, in pretending. Although it would be dreamlike.

MAY 24

I don't take any shit anymore. All of a sudden it is identifiable and, therefore, avoidable or extractable.

Don't give her no shit, she won't take it. She doesn't eat shit anymore. She doesn't even want it in the same room anymore.

Jobs, even jobs, are quitable.

People are leavable when they're shitdishers.

Shit's easily digestible when you can't see it.

When you see it, all of a sudden you don't want any part of it.

Why did I ever take it? And why won't I take it anymore?

JUNE 6

"You can't start a fire without a spark," sing it, Bruce, I'm listening now to that classic song of yours.

Just a spark these days. Burning. Flaring. Young and full of lust and love and adventure.

My body wants to be filled all the time. I'm young and fit from the long walks and hungry, and full of a delicious actor. Did I ever tell you that sex is great?

It truly is. Laugh and pooh-pooh at the past. This is it, baby. And there's so much more out there.

The artist as a young woman.

JULY 2

I want to be twenty-two forever.

Josh Levine has fallen in love with me.

Grreat.

Today, I loved him being in love with me.

The actor not acting is superb.

Now is all. No more.

All's fine.

All's well.

Sarah's my friend.

Tonight, my cup runneth over.

OXOXOXOX

JULY 7

1:24 A.M.

I do not just want to be young, old, and die.

I do not want to need anybody. I don't want to cry and want and need.

Josh said he loves me and that took me in. I don't want to need.

How does it all work?

Where is everyone now that school is out for the summer?

I've been crying a lot more lately.

I may have decided to leave it, but it still remains that the TV newsroom is all gone.

Lisa Messinger
Newsroom
1-1-1-1

EVERYTHING YOU ALWAYS WANTED TO KNOW ABOUT TELEVISION NEWS, BUT WERE AFRAID TO ASK

"This is not a glamorous job," the manager of news operations told me as I sat stuck to the vinyl chair in his cubicle of an office in the newsroom at KDUM, a leading independent station in a major western city. As I took note of the large cardboard file boxes marked "resumes" stacked from floor to ceiling against the west wall of the room, I said I didn't want glamour, just an opportunity to work in a television newsroom.

Well, glamour was about as far from life at KDUM as was a forty share of ratings for their evening newscast. Whenever I think about those boxes of resumes, I can't help but wonder if those thousands of broadcasting, communications, and journalism graduates from Maine to South Carolina to Kansas knew how lucky they were to receive the standard KDUM "Sorry No Vacancy" letter. Would they be lucky enough, I wondered, to turn to real estate or paralegal work or perhaps managing a Kentucky Fried Chicken store?

I, needless to say, was not. I took the production assistant job for which the human resources department hinted over 4,000 people had applied. It is my intention here to paint a picture of life in the television newsroom (I have a network of friends at other stations, who lead me to believe that, give or take a few ratings points, things are pretty much the same all over). It's a friendly warning to beginners, and a reference guide for all others who ever wondered what more there is to television news besides ratings.

First of all, let's dispel a myth. Beginners do not really need a journalism degree. This is just used as a tool to weed out the hundreds of thousands of other people who would apply for the jobs if the actual skills were really known. Let me, for perhaps the first time in print, set down the true prerequisites for most entry-level broadcasting positions.

1) **Waitressing or waitering experience.** The production assistant or messenger or go-fer, or whatever the station chooses to call its hired servant, must be able to take dinner orders with the proficiency of a skilled, seasoned waiter. There is no end, for example, to the variations on the theme of, let's say, a corned beef sandwich. There's, of course, your standard corned beef on rye with mustard. There is also, however, corned beef with mayo on whole wheat, corned beef on white toast with alfalfa sprouts, corned beef on Armenian bread with green peppers, and a personal favorite of one KDUM writer, Chinese corned beef chicken salad.

Although orders often come from such varied locales as McDonald's, Bernie's Vegetarian Garden, and Gustav's Goulash Palace, KDUM messengers are expected to do dinner runs in no more than twelve minutes. Once when an order of chicken paprika was held up at Gustav's because it was being specially deboned for our director Henny Sleinball, it took me sixteen minutes to get back to the station. Since two writers had already fallen face down onto their typewriters and the producer was forced to resort to cold Spaghettios from the KDUM vending machine, I was told to go straight to the corner and rip copy from the wire machines without my Big Mac dinner.

2) Professional race car driving experience.

This is on a par in importance with restaurant experience. Having driven in the Indianapolis 500 or at Daytona would certainly be something to list before *New York Times* or *Washington Post* stringer experience on your resume. When KDUM couriers are hired, they are given an official KDUM bumper sticker that says, "Yes, that's right, I do own the whole damn road," and tips on such important things as how to easily spot highway patrolmen, and how to most effectively place your "News Media" placard on the dashboard for easy identification.

The correct placement of the "News Media" sign can become crucial at certain times. Take parking situations. When it becomes necessary to park on sidewalks, in hotel lobbies, or on top of other vehicles, it is important to have the sign properly displayed.

Couriers, on the other hand, do have some KDUM rules by which they must abide. They are not under any circumstances allowed to drive over 120 miles per hour (it could hurt the car), and they are warned against driving through intersections while more than six pedestrians are crossing (lawsuits can be costly).

While professional race car driving and waitering experience is important job preparation for aspiring newsroom applicants, there are certain academic prerequisites that should not be missed. Be sure to take the basic first aid or introductory pre-med class. This will come in handy on the many occasions you will get stabbed in the back. Make

sure, also, that you read the classics *Looking Out for Number One* and *How to Be Your Own Best Friend*. It's just as important, too, not to miss the screening of "All About Eve" in the introductory cinema course. As most newsroom beginners will tell you, this kind of knowledge is invaluable.

It's too bad that KiKi Carlyse, an aspiring KDUM anchor, didn't know her abc's when it came to backstabbing. She believed Rochelle Rodanski, another aspiring anchor, when she told her a message had come in saying her grandmother had accidentally fallen out of a seven-story building and broken her hip. KiKi rushed to the hospital, and Rochelle, who was at that time an unpaid intern, valiantly took over her duties, telling Art Belchco, manager of news operations, that she thought it was about time he knew about KiKi's fiendish and uncontrollable cocaine habit.

As well as classes that should be taken, there are classes that it would be more helpful than not to miss. Do not, for example, take anything based on Dale Carnegie's *How to Make Friends and Influence People,* avoid all communications classes, and do not take philosophy courses, especially logic or ethics.

It was harder, for example, for anyone at KDUM who had taken logic or ethics to understand why Marc Hereditarian was promoted than it was for people without these backgrounds. Marc came into the KDUM newsroom as a janitor. However, within two days, he was a seven-figure-a-year KDUM golden-jacketed sportscaster. Later, we found out that he was a friend of KDUM chairman of the board Carl Beefsky's lawyer's barber's son.

I shouldn't paint the newsroom experience, however, as such a completely harrowing one. I do think I remember that Melvin Bean, KDUM anchorman, did on one occasion thank me for my nightly carrying of his fifty-pound full-length mirror over to the news set. And if my memory serves me correctly, KDUM news executive producer Gordon Tinkle did once promise that if I ever worked six consecutive eighty-hour weeks again, I might see a bonus in my paycheck of two Drive-In Monster Movie Marathon tickets for our local theatre.

Well, I never received that bonus. I walked out of the KDUM door that reads, "If it's News, it's News to Us," for the last time about two months ago. I now work as a freelance writer during the day, and, at night, in order to make ends meet, I work part time as a waitress at Gustav's Goulash Palace. As I debone chicken each night for the weary-looking KDUM messenger, I think that what my new job lacks in glamour, at least it makes up for in tips.

JULY 19

Twenty-two-and-a-half inches. Do you believe it? Do you believe it? Twenty-two-and-a-half inches—*TV Guide,* the most read publication in the nation, wrote twenty-two-and-a-half inches on the copy of my TV news article they returned. They inched out my article! This place that I wondered if they would even read my article, took the time to determine how much space my article would fill on the hallowed pages of *TV Guide.* It would have filled twenty-two-and-a-half inches, I would have been paid, and it would have been read all over the country. Their note said they too recently had run an article with a slightly similar theme. Damn.

SEPTEMBER 7

I love finally knowing where things are in New York. It's hard to believe Sarah and I were just in the city I had dreamed about so much. Now, when I read and a place is mentioned, I can halfway picture it. I count out streets, I think Uptown, Midtown, Downtown, the Lower East Side, the West side.

I see the city on film, in video, and I know it. I know the mystery now, but have I solved it? Will it take another trip, will it take more?

Four months 'til graduation is a short burp. Four months is enough to scare you out of your wits if you let the top off. Four months is enough. Four years, on the other hand, is beginning to seem like four months just short of enough. Enough of a major independent TV station. Enough of a major metropolitan city, although I am a hummer, for sure, of "I Love L.A."

SEPTEMBER 8

I went into school knowing exactly what I wanted to do, wanting only to finally be able to do it. I come out of school not sure of what to choose, knowing only the sad truth, the utter reality, of a certain few dreams. Which are left? Which will do? Enough money, the right hours, but what of enough challenge, enough adventure, the eventual contribution? I never thought I would lose that desire, but I guess everybody says that. I still want to believe and hope that I may be different, that I am different. I'm just not sure anymore.

SEPTEMBER 10

Why am I so goddamned jealous of Sarah? It's not that I'm really even jealous—envious, I mean—not really wishing that I was doing what she was doing, not wishing that I was making x-hundred dollars a week while still a student (her full-time TV newsroom pay is certainly a lot more than my part-time TV station pay!), not wishing that I was doing all kinds of exciting things in my chosen profession. Really, I'm not jealous. I'm just upset. This gnawing feeling tells me not to want to listen to my roommate's day at work, to the stories that last year used to make my mind perk.

She has money, and I don't. She has somehow leaped ahead of me. I was always ahead of everyone. Now there's someone so clearly ahead, and my roommate, my perhaps best friend. It's hard to live with such drive. I feel that I have drive, but it's on hold. It's hard to have drive and eighteen units and twenty hours of work all in the same week.

Like I said, I don't think I should be in that place now. I don't even want to be. I don't want to be on such a set path already. I like having dabbled, and dabbling in lots of related things. I write. I program. I newsed. I documentaried. I paged. I don't want to be pegged. But, somehow, because she's already working in broadcast journalism as an assistant producer and seems so sure of exactly what she wants to do, I feel the pressure breathing down my neck. We're so comparable, and she's making money in a field where the pay is supposed to be dirt. She's pretty obviously going to make it.

Sometimes, I don't even feel like I know where I'm going anymore. That's what I guess is so distressing. There seems like so many things I could do, and I feel terror at making the wrong choice, even though I know, at this early point, there aren't that many wrong choices.

Well, I have very important classes this last time, and I know I want to *be* there, not obsessed with audition tapes, and resumés and all. I know this stuff is important, and it's the last time.

I know I still have every opportunity to be everything I ever thought I could be. I know I'm not even out of college yet. I know I'm a published author. I know if I had talent, I still have talent. I know that I'm not really behind, but in the right place for me. It's still easy, however, to feel threatened—aware at what seems like too many moments, just how human I am. Did I really used to be an angel?

SEPTEMBER 15

How human do I have to be? Is this a test, or what? Really, I know I'm human. This is completely unnecessary. I don't need a pending romance between my roommate and Mr. Desirable flaunted in front of my face.

Why is he punching her? What's wrong with me, I'm not good enough to punch? Why does he have to be so handsome? So sharp? So built? Why does he have to live next door? Why does he have to punch my roommate?

Aren't I pretty? Does this mean that her personality so outweighs mine that it blocks it out? "Friendly" is her middle name, is it not? First and last, too. But that's my attraction to her also, so I can see it.

Of course, he's much more attractive to both of us because the picture holds three. He's not immediately my type, but are we in some kind of contest now? She's ahead, isn't she?

How did I always win before? Why can't I have whatever I want?

This is a test. I know it. Only a test of the emergency broadcast system. If this were a real emergency you would be told where to tune for news and information.

SEPTEMBER 22

Saturday Night
I am having an affair. The kind in the movies. And with an actor, by coincidence. I am writing a book, the kind that gets published, in fact.

Josh looks great in a towel. And I am delirious, in fact. Tell me, how did I get what seems to be the best combination ever of every tall, dark, and handsome actor who ever lived, in my bed?

In my bed. That's where we've been. In my bed.

Eight months. Peaking. Peaking, yes we are. An actor's in love with me. And I am peaking. All the while.

SEPTEMBER 25

All of a sudden it hits you, like when you realize you're in love with a friend you've known for a long time. All of sudden, there's passion, and fire, and you know what was so obvious all along, what was meant to be.

It was obvious, all the pieces were there, and you never saw what was right in front of you. The blank page. You're going to be a writer after all, aren't you?

SEPTEMBER 27

What happens when you might get a book published? It's hard to concentrate on anything except for the fact that your words might be bound and pressed forever. Go to school? Ha! Ha! Sit still? Ha. The infinite possibility that is in the publisher's hand. To make you immortal, no matter how few know. Immortal, no matter how long it stays in print, because you would have a copy to pass on. The dream. The dream of the writer.

But what of the fledgling? The unpublished? What of her? What excitement. The answer, the key. The start of her imminent, long-awaited career.

What of her? Is it going to happen to her?

OCTOBER 1

12:30 A.M.

I fell in love. I didn't try, and I don't know how it happened. But I guess it did. It doesn't matter where we go or what we do, it's eclectic or electric or just wow! Everyone says that, but it's true.

I think I love Josh. Did he ask me if I'd ever thought of living in New York? Yes. And I thought it at that moment. Us two in a loft, an artist's studio, a little apartment. Writing. Acting. We said we'd keep each other warm.

Just a thought. But I begin to like the sight of him more and more. And certainly the feel. And definitely the sound. I'm a woman in love. With all her options open.

OCTOBER 2

I'm walking around in a daze because it's not a dream anymore, it's real. The thing that was just a dream a month ago is now beginning to seem real. Plans are not dreams. Details are not dreams. Book publishers' calls are not dreams. Talk of money is not a dream. This thing I thought was my ultimate dream choice to do when I finished school is now as real as anything else. Why is it that my dreams always come true?

Advice for the Rest of Your Life

We are about to end our journey together. Today Lisa leads a wonderful life, a life full of meaning: love, friendships, success, and the fulfillment of so many of her diary dreams. The journey for Lisa has not always been an easy one and has taken unexpected twists and turns, but her determination to overcome her life-threatening eating disorder has taken her to a far better place. You are now on the road to recovery. Congratulations—it is not an easy place to be, but like Lisa, your determination, strength, and the supports you are seeking will see you through. As you read this chapter and the last chapters of Lisa's diary, perhaps you will find insights to make the final steps toward long-term health and happiness a little easier, as you, too, move toward realizing your dreams.

THE BIG "R"—RELAPSE

Let's move back for a moment to Chapter 10, *Promises, Promises*. What was happening there is very important. Lisa was on her way to recovery. Her life was improving, she had come to the vital realization that this was not only about food and body size, and her insights were coming at a rapid pace. Just when we think that all is well, just when Lisa tells us she will never binge again, something completely unexpected happens to change the picture. That something is called relapse. Lisa makes a decision to stop binging, and for two weeks all is well. Then, in an unexpected turn, she begins a starvation diet, goes back to thinking of food as "good" and "bad," and begins to again eat in secret as she isolates more and more. She again writes about the disruption in her relationships being caused by her weight. We, as readers, are able to see what Lisa cannot. Her eating disorder is beginning to again regain control. This is called relapse.

A Normal Part of Recovery

As you move toward recovery, relapses can and will happen. Unfortunately, they are frequently a part of recovery. It is important to remember that, even though your eating disorder was quite possibly life threatening, in many ways it may have served a vital and protective purpose. Often, an eating disorder helps mask feelings of pain, rejection, sadness, loneliness, sexual confusions, boredom, disappointment, spiritual emptiness, past traumas, and family turmoil. As this was occurring, all that you were aware of is that as you manipulated your eating, you sometimes briefly felt a little better. Often, you felt numb. In any case, the feelings were temporarily contained. The key word is temporarily, because, as you are now learning, the feelings were only shelved to return at a later date with renewed intensity as the unresolved problems festered and grew. Life for all of us can at times be hard, and we are all sometimes overwhelmed with very intense and difficult feelings that involve past and future, as well as present events. It is at these times that you probably will return to thoughts of food, excessive exercise, and body control as a means of coping. As your therapy progresses, however, you will learn new and better ways to deal with these complex feelings that do not involve a return to old eating disorder patterns.

When my daughter, Stephanie, was five, she taught me an important lesson. She had a bad ski fall and I went to pick her up. The small child looked up at her worried mom calmly and said, "Mom, I'm okay. It's not how hard you fall but how you get up." So remember, relapse happens. It's not how hard you fall but how you get up. Your task is to get up and start again. You can do it!

Know the Signals

Know the signals. It is important to view relapse as a learning experience. Although relapse may seem to occur without warning, in reality the spiraling events that lead to relapse frequently have a pattern. If you can learn that pattern, that is, understand your unique signals, you can catch a relapse in the early stages when it is much easier to turn around. Let's look for a minute at Lisa.

Lisa's relapses frequently had to do with relationships with men, the primary relationship being with her father. "Another gray area involves my dad," Lisa writes. "On the surface everything's peachy, but I find myself feeling very mad and frustrated about him. When I came back from Palm Springs he blew up at me for no reason. . . . He said he didn't like my attitude or the type of person I was becoming. . . . He asked me how I thought he felt when he saw me ten to fifteen pounds heavier. . . . I didn't even do anything." Lisa's feelings of being not loved unconditionally, and undervalued, by her father were an important part of her therapeutic work and pivotal in understanding her eating disorder. Comments about weight and body size from her father were particularly painful. In addition, as Lisa began to change, her father had difficulty adjusting to the new Lisa, and conflicts with her family became an important relapse trigger.

Romantic relationships provided other relapse triggers for Lisa. Throughout her journal, rejection or sometimes just perceived rejection from men led to relapse, even though other men were also complimenting her and trying to woo her. Surprisingly, love and acceptance from men she deeply cared about also led to relapse. We see this clearly when Bob arrives and professes his love for Lisa, triggering an intense desire to eat, and in her serious close relationship with David, which just goes to show that stress, whether caused for "good" or "bad" reasons, can be a relapse trigger. A deeper look might also show that Lisa's fear of being loved, and also fear of her increasing sexual feelings, may have led to the relapse, as she accurately noted in her journal (as her own ability to identify relapse triggers increased). Nonetheless, what is most important to note is that strong emotion, either positive or negative, may be a relapse trigger.

Lisa's sexual feelings and desires also caused her internal conflict and were a powerful relapse trigger. "I've discovered in the past few days . . . that I like sex. I really like it. Maybe that's connected to the "stuffing" I've been doing. My feelings and actions in the past regarding sex have been pretty ambivalent. The past three weeks, the past few days, really, have been the first time I really ever truly let go, just feel and listen to my body. (I didn't even know my body could tell me such things.)" Just as Lisa is learning to value and appreciate her sexual feelings she is learning to value, appreciate, and trust her body in a far different way that has nothing to do with body weight and food. She is learning to feel her body.

Since each and every one of you is unique and special, the triggers for relapse will be different. Your signals may have to do with rejection or perceived rejection, pain, sadness, loneliness, exhaustion, boredom, or disappointment, or a host of other feelings. As you become more and more aware of your feelings in therapy, the signals will become clearer and you will find yourself aware of them at a much earlier stage. Old thinking patterns, as well as the belief in eating disorder fairy tales and myths, die hard. Do not be surprised if they return to haunt you well into the recovery process. In fact, for many years to come, when under extreme pressures, there may be a part of you that thinks about running for comfort to your old patterns. "It felt right to feel sick again over food. Like, welcome home. Comfortable. Like I've been away for a long time, but come back to the warmth, the numbness. Come back to where it doesn't hurt (on the surface) anymore. Come back. Come back. Come back," Lisa wrote less than a year into her therapy. Lisa had some relapses, but she continued to bravely struggle, just as you will, growing and gaining control of her eating disorder and of her life.

"I'm not going to fall back into the isolation. I'm not going to cut myself off from My World. I'm not going to crawl back into my yellow wallpapered shell with the rose-colored trim," Lisa wrote. "God, I'm getting beckoned again, though. But do I have to go? Succumb? Retreat? No, No, No. No, No,

No. In fact, No Way. I can keep going, keep moving, keep the circulation going. I can listen to the directions from the cynic in me with one ear so that I can move with both feet in the opposite direction!" This time around, you, like Lisa, can be more aware of the early warning signals of relapse as you, too, take control of your eating disorder and of your life.

SEEKING SUPPORT

At this point, you may be feeling proud of your progress on the road to recovery and you may feel, as you should, more in control. You may even believe that if you identify the relapse signals early enough you can handle the situation alone. In addition, the same stressors that lead to relapse may lead to another old but very familiar pattern—isolation. Do not isolate! No matter how independent you are, periods of potential relapse are the times that you will need the most support. Lisa's relapse occurred when she stopped seeing her individual therapist and group therapy ended. All of her most important supports were no longer there. The letters from Jane, one of the members in her support group, helped turn things around as they proved an important form of support, just as Jane also commented how Lisa's letters helped her tremendously.

Support can come in many forms. You can and should continue seeing your therapist as long as is necessary. Don't stop too soon. Your therapist or support group can provide much needed help. Lisa confided in me that, although what she learned in therapy kept her out of the trap of an eating disorder from then onward, she probably stopped therapy too early due to her father's cutting it off and her own feeling of thinking she was quite a bit improved. She never even knew of the additional safeguards that can be taken, the aftercare, etc., until we talked years later in preparing this book. She feels that some of the bumps along the way afterward, especially in recognizing and dealing with stress and reaching out for support rather than isolating herself, could have been further improved with additional therapy at the time.

Therefore, don't be shy about staying in touch with your support team. When you feel you need to, for instance, contact your nutritionist or other professionals with whom you have worked. Even if you have not seen them for a period of time, they will usually try to be available. Reach out to family members, friends, religious or spiritual leaders, or groups or community groups like OA. Consider writing a list of your support people with their contact information in advance and put it in an easily accessible place. The most important thing is to reach out. There will be others there to help and to get you back on track. In turn, at a later time, with all of the knowledge you have gained, you will be there to help others on their journey, just as Lisa has done.

REEXAMINING OLD THINKING PATTERNS— REVISITING FAIRY TALES AND MYTHS

As you recover, you probably will be surprised to find how much your eating disorder has distorted your thinking and perceptions. You may also be surprised to find out how much of the way you view the world around you is changing. For Lisa, major changes came in her black-and-white approach to the world. In the early chapters of her diary, her friendships, love relationships, school, and job, indeed, the whole world around her, was either the best or the worst. This is a very difficult way to live and the constant emotional ups and downs associated with this way of thinking are sure setups for a binge. Black-and-white thinking was particularly evident in her food choices. Most people with eating disorders see food choices as either good or bad. As a result, most fat-, carbohydrate-, or calorie-dense food becomes forbidden, not only creating a severe nutritional imbalance, but also setting up fertile ground for obsessing about the forbidden food, and binging. In later recovery, Lisa writes, "Things don't have to be *either* wonderful *or* awful anymore. There is an in between. I know because I'm in it right now, and it's so much easier than the *burden* of each extreme."

Closely allied to this black-and-white thinking was Lisa's need to be perfect and to be the best, not only the best body size and weight, but also to have the best boyfriend and the best job. Her intense drive led her to very early career success, but the price was enormous. You, too, may feel that you must be perfect in everything that you do. It might be useful during your recovery to examine how this pattern developed. Do you, like Lisa, feel that you have to be perfect to be loved? Does perfectionism frequently center around your body and weight? You, like Lisa, will begin to realize that your quest for perfectionism, in an imperfect and sometimes unpredictable world, is just not possible, and that it is really just a setup for pain. You, like Lisa, will begin to discover that you are a human being and not a human doing; that you are worthy and special, deserving to give, and increasingly receive, love, even if you are imperfect.

Let's look briefly at a few of the fairy tales. In reexamining these myths and fairy tales, you will find that they are merely that—myths and fairy tales— and this discovery will negate any power over you that they have had. Although I will touch on only two of the fairy tales as examples, upon rereading pages 86–92, you will probably find that the others have also begun to change.

Fairy Tale One: I am in control. As you move along your road to recovery, one of the most surprising things you probably have discovered is that you were never really in control at all. During this period, your eating disorder had always been in control, and in battles, the eating disorder won each and every time. We watch as Lisa struggles and increasingly gains real control of the

world around her. "You know what it was, though, *fear* and way too much control over myself. Well, it's funny what happened, I let down my guard, and let
myself be natural. I'm not scared anymore, and I feel I've gained more real control (not the artificial kind I had before)," she wrote. As you progress in your
therapy, you will become more and more aware of the fears, feelings, and old
issues that make you feel you need control. You will also become more aware
of the areas of your life in which you do have control and more able to "go
with the flow" in areas that you do not. You, like Lisa, will become more and
more aware of your internal personal power.

Fairy Tale Two: I will be popular. At this point you have probably found,
like Lisa, that initially thinness did bring increased attention. You may have
attracted more members of the opposite sex and very briefly felt more special.
This, however, was probably short lived, since the eating disorder began to
take over and with it feelings of shame, guilt, and low self-esteem. A world
centered around food and exercise replaced any feeling of being special. In this
isolated world, new relationships and friendships became difficult to maintain
and you may have ended up largely alone.

Lisa writes about this harsh reality in what I believe is one of the most
important parts of her diary, and she recognizes it almost immediately afterward, too: "The vision of a murderess had been brewing in my mind for a long
time, ever since I gradually started gaining back the weight I had lost in the
summer after my high school graduation. That was when for a few months I
turned into the beautiful, happy, skinny, very popular girl I had always
dreamed of being. . . . What I finally realized that day [in the psychologist's
office] as she had me role-play the part of the beautiful happy thin dead girl
was that I had not really been happy then. I had been a robot, a beautiful,
popular, skinny *robot*. I neither really thought nor felt during that time. . . . My
life had not been filled with the happiness I now chose to believe it had been
filled with. Instead, it was filled, and completely saturated, with control, regimented diet, exercise, and even dating schedules. I wasn't free, I was like a
machine. That day was the first time I cried in her office. . . . I felt a wave of
self-acceptance come over me that was different than any other such feeling I
had experienced while in therapy."

These are just a few of the myths and fairy tales Lisa eradicated forever
while in therapy. You will surely be as excited and relieved as she was as you
begin to do the same. As you recover, you may be surprised how the "true"
you draws friendship, intimacy, and love based on the unique person you are
inside—not on body weight and size.

NEW RELATIONSHIPS

Lisa has begun to reestablish relationships with girlfriends and with people at
work and at school. "One of the things I've realized, and it's been tough, is the

value of real friends. I was lonely because I cut myself off from everyone for so long, and they didn't know why. . . . Right now, I feel like I'm rebuilding everything."

"Nourishing myself is what I'm doing. I can see it at work. I am being nourished by the friendship and experience of the older (somewhat) women. Being nourished at home by the young spirit of the college co-eds I call wondrous to be around. Nourished by my family, my friends. For all the nourishing I did, only to end up malnourished and dehydrated."

For so long, Lisa's primary relationship has been with food. That is now changing, leaving ample room for the nourishment of relationships with people. "I am flourishing as an individual. And within that flourishing, I can be nourished and cherished by those who surround me."

Lisa's relationship with her father (through much work in therapy and far greater understanding on both of their parts) has changed. There is a greater level of understanding, more comfort on being together, and the all-essential ability to just talk. We are reminded over and over in these chapters just how much Lisa's relationship with men has changed.

She is far more in touch with her feelings and desires. Even more importantly, she feels better about herself and realizes that she now has the ability to choose and not just wait to be chosen. She also realizes that she no longer has to perform and be what the men she is with expect. "Then during this newer relationship with David, right from the beginning, I had a different attitude. . . . For once, I just let myself be. I didn't make it a reward or a condition or make its happening depend on other things (like losing weight or something else) happening first. I just let it (no made it) happen to me. And felt it was the best thing I'd ever done." She has learned, in regard to her relationships with men, to be herself.

In fact, she has been happily married for quite a few years to the actor she describes in her last diary chapters! Her true nourishment is coming from people and not food. These relationships were an important part of her road to recovery.

FEELINGS, NOT FOOD

Like Lisa, you are probably already becoming aware of the fact that your eating disorder is really more about feelings than food. Common emotional triggers for binging or restricting include pain, fear, competition, jealousy, loneliness, abandonment, and anger. No matter what the feelings, you, like Lisa, may have found that large quantities of certain foods seemed to make the feelings disappear as if by magic, leaving a temporary sense of calm and relief from the powerful emotions. For a brief time you may have even imagined that the food made you happy. Unfortunately, though, the "food happy" feeling was fleeting and frequently followed by periods of shame, guilt, and renewed retreats into binging or restricting.

By masking all of these difficult feelings, often for years, nothing was resolved or understood. The feelings didn't disappear, but were put on a temporary shelf only to return at a later time, creating renewed internal chaos. A good example of this lies in Lisa's struggles with her sexuality. Repression of her growing sexual feelings and needs created confusion, chaos, and relapse. Acknowledging and accepting these powerful feelings allowed Lisa to make important life decisions and aided her on her road to recovery.

The role of fear and anxiety is particularly important in the development of an eating disorder. It is important to realize that fear and anxiety have promoted many of your eating-disordered behaviors as self-protective mechanisms. To let go of these self-protective behaviors is to take a big risk. To let go of these behaviors means to fully and completely allow yourself to feel, and this is not an easy task. Your eating disorder had previously helped you to block feelings. It is important, at this time, that you not retreat from the powerful feelings that will emerge during your recovery. Some of these feelings have been masked for a long time. Your therapist, group, or nutritionist can help you to better understand the often-confusing internal cues that are occurring as you learn and grow. It is important to remember that the urge to binge and purge or restrict may not go away for a long period of time and any period of intense feeling, at least in the early stages of recovery, may make you want to retreat to old eating-disordered behaviors. Like Lisa, this is one thing that you will continue to fight against as you move forward. However, you will become more and more adept at recognizing, accepting, and dealing with feelings. In fact, a greater understanding of your feelings will be a significant asset in successfully navigating your life's path.

DEVELOPING A HEALTHY RELATIONSHIP WITH FOOD

Healthy eating means eating when you are hungry, eating what is good for your body and also what you want, and stopping when you have had enough. It means enjoying the taste, texture, and smell of food. It has to do with pleasure in shopping for food, cooking, and eating with others. It has to do with eating to satisfy bodily, and not emotional, needs for nurturance. Perhaps equally important, it has to do with eating beyond the point of fullness once in a while because you love the taste of what you are eating, or it is a special occasion, without feeling shame or guilt. Healthy eating has to do with respecting your body and its unique needs.

Although this may seem basic, if you have been living with an eating disorder for a long time, you may have forgotten what healthy eating is. You may know surprisingly little about satiety (knowing when you are physically full) and hunger. You may no longer trust, or often be unaware of, your own body cues, telling you when you are hungry and need to eat and when you are full. Often you may not know what you want to eat partly because so many of the foods you most like have been "forbidden," and stopping when you are full may feel almost impossible. There may be little pleasure in shopping for or cooking food for yourself, although you may be a wonderful cook when it comes to others. Eating with others may have been a purposely rare occasion. Although food may be calming and soothing, it is less often associated with pleasure than with shame and guilt. The wonderful news is that as you develop a healthy relationship with food, all of these things will most likely change.

Some people, particularly in the early stages of recovery, find a structured meal plan, developed with the help of your nutritionist, to be useful. Dr. Mowey Mohafy, a well-respected nutritionist, says that meal plans can be an effective way to provide the necessary structure and security that allows his clients to trust themselves to consume an adequate amount of food. In the early stages of recovery you may be unable to trust your own feelings of hunger and fullness, you will not be sure of your body's healthy food needs, and, most importantly, you will be terrified of gaining weight. Your new meal plan can teach you food and eating habits that will help to keep you healthy (not fat) and strong. Mohafy continues, "Letting go of food rules and rituals, improving variety and adequacy of food intake, and addressing misconceptions about nutrition and weight can all be a part of the process of using meal plans."

We clearly see this with Lisa near the end of her diary. Gone are the lists of binge foods and the notations of the calorie counts of every morsel that goes into her mouth. Gone are the writings of anguish about breaking her ironclad control over the food she eats. Lisa is not obsessed with food any longer; that is obvious. Instead, her writing is bubbling with the excitement of meeting new friends, romantic partners, and new and challenging jobs, like that in the television newsroom. She has learned to eat nutritiously for fuel: "My God, I didn't even try to lose weight. It's just that going to school in the morning, working four hours in the TV station programming department in the afternoon, and working three nights a week in the TV newsroom left only time to eat for energy."

Getting back on track can be difficult, but it will help to remember some basic guidelines. What you are seeking is total health and well-being rather than an "ideal" weight at any cost. Lisa was surprised, as we read, when this dawned on her during therapy. Humans are diverse in regard to size and weight. Respect your own diversity. You were born with a certain genetic weight range and may never look like the models in a magazine. What you will look like is a healthy and beautiful you. It is more important to respect your internal cues of hunger and fullness rather than external plans and diets. Remember flexibility, balance, variety, moderation, and respect for your unique needs.

RECLAIMING THE MURDERED SELF

Lisa first brought up her "murdered self" in conjunction with the eradication of her "fairy tale" thinking patterns, but, for her and probably you, that is just the beginning when it comes to the essential reclaiming of your true murdered self (not the "once-thin" person you got rid of, but the "real" person you had banished). For far too long, your eating disorder probably has caused you to lose the essential you. You are on the road to recovery and all of that is changing. You have rediscovered the fact that you are much more than your body and your weight. You are a unique and special person who no longer depends on the love and approval of others to feel good about yourself. "I realized that all of the things that made me realize I was happy had solely to do with me, stemmed just from me. The people who are helping make my life full now are my people. . . . My job decisions. Actual decisions. My advances toward that special one of the opposite sex." "I really am controlling my life. It's not just happening through someone else," Lisa triumphantly wrote. You have hopefully become more and more aware of the many strengths that lie inside. You have begun to reclaim your murdered self.

Through therapy, the help of others, and sometimes painful self-examination, Lisa began to truly reclaim her murdered self. "I know who I am and what I want, and anything I do is not changing that. I'm proud of myself, not for blatantly external achievements, but for the way I'm grappling with these personal issues." "Of course, there must be some way things could be better, and things could certainly be worse, but I wouldn't trade places with anyone at all," she wrote. Lisa worked on her relationship with her father, and both have grown in the process. She has sought more in-depth and growth-producing love relationships, all the while becoming more comfortable with and more appreciative of her sexual feelings. When we leave Lisa she has begun a very special relationship with the man she will later marry. More significantly, relationships with women, like her relationship with Jane, help to complete the picture. Lisa has learned to reach out and to let people in.

As her diary closes, Lisa has come a long way from the weight- and calorie-obsessed young teen she was. She came to grips with her weight and began to love and care for the genetic body she had been given. "You know something, I just realized I still weigh 140 pounds," she wrote. "And you know what, weight doesn't even matter to me anymore." This is the same Lisa who wanted to weigh 103 pounds to the exclusion of every single one of her true human needs. As Lisa recovered from her eating disorder, her weight dropped, seemingly without effort, to 130 pounds, close to her genetically determined weight. To her surprise, Lisa writes, "I weigh 130 pounds and last night, Josh, a man (special!) was telling me what a great body I have."

Lisa has also come to appreciate her strengths and abilities in a far more in-depth and real way than the constant empty and almost frantic mani-festations we saw in the earlier chapters. Finally, we see Lisa realizing her dream—to be a writer. What is most interesting is that we can almost track Lisa's recovery through her writing style. Toward the end of the diary, the ini-tially light articles become confident and opinionated as she becomes more and more aware of how she thinks and feels.

You, too, hopefully are, or can soon be, on the road to recovery. What are your gifts and talents? What are the very special things that make you unique? For many of my clients in the early stages of recovery, this is a very difficult question to answer, and so I suggest an assignment. Perhaps you would like to try the same assignment. Buy any kind of notebook and some simple art supplies. You are about to design your own affirmation book. On the cover put your name and any drawing or design that represents you. This is your affirmation book and each day you will write something you like about yourself, something you are proud of, or a new insight or step in your recov-ery in the book. So many new and exciting things will be happening and you will be feeling better and better about yourself. Basically, what you will be doing each day is affirming yourself, that is, developing more and more awareness of your uniqueness and increasing strength. In addition, I suggest sharing the book on a regular basis with family, friends, or your support group. Let others write their affirmations of you. Don't be afraid to ask. It's really fun. On a more serious level, during difficult or stressful times—and there will most likely always be tough times in your recovery—pull out your book and read. You may find this very simple book becomes a treasured friend. Lisa has told me she has done this a number of times over the years with her diary, and it's been of tremendous therapeutic help to her, seeming to help her in a unique way each time she reads it.

We have shared a long journey together. In closing, Lisa writes: "That past, though, is becoming less and less of a burden to haul around. It lives on in the pages of this journal It lives on, too, in a little corner of my mind. There's no rent control, though, in that particular corner. The rates for staying on keep getting higher and higher. Few of those old-timers can afford to pay, so they're packing up and moving out, leaving room for newer, more amiable tenants." Lisa remains in recovery. "No matter what happens in my life, something must stay constant, a feeling of self-validation, the feeling of satisfaction with self. No matter what, this must *be*." Her life is productive and happy. On many lev-els she has fulfilled so many of her dreams.

You may be just beginning your journey, but it is not too soon to begin to look ahead and dream about where you, too, are heading. Like Lisa, you are beginning to truly value your own uniqueness, special gifts, and most of all courage. Now is your time to dream of new directions and your new life, free of the shackles of your eating disorder. Remember—it's not how you fall but how you get up that counts. I have enjoyed sharing the journey with you. Continue to always reach out. You are not alone!

Epilogue

I asked in the final line of my last journal entry, "Why is it that my dreams always come true?" Well, clearly, it takes a long time for some dreams to come true. It takes a clear, unencumbered, uncluttered mind. I realized, for example, that, although someday my journalism career might naturally bring me into the realm of broadcast journalism, that I did not have that "need" to be on camera, that I could be happy as—and, indeed, my first choice was to be—a writer or print reporter. It was part of my old, shy, closed-up, insecure personality that had needed the attention and recognition that comes through television. Now, I just naturally have these things in my real life and don't "need" to seek them in a career.

I also don't need what I used to from my father. You'll notice he is not mentioned much in the last part of this journal. That's because, after the initial therapeutic explosion between us, I was already nineteen years old. Legally, an adult. When he started gradually to read about bulimia, see my psychologist on TV, or hear her on radio and tell me about what he learned, I thought, "It's too late, Buddy. You missed your chance. Here I am, I am grown up, and you lost me to another man, my all-loving David."

Clearly, I was still hurt. However, when the all-loving David broke off with me, devastated, I went home many weekends to my parents' home. And I was surprised. I knew I'd get support from my mom. She'd call him every name in the book and be on my side. But, deep down, I thought my dad would think David was right, I should be left, I was not good enough to marry, I should try and get this intelligent, successful male back.

Well, at this very crucial point for me, I got sincere support and understanding and sympathy from my father. He felt that I was young and had everything going for me, and David wasn't right for me, and there was nothing at all wrong with me. He said, although maybe there was a sixty percent chance we would get back together, maybe we shouldn't.

At present, I wouldn't hesitate talking about anything at all with either of my parents. And I often do. My mom always understands. My dad many times does. I am now, however, more than aware that he cares about me, all parts of me, not just the brain and the outer crust.

And, even though I was already nineteen years old when that all happened, it wasn't too late to intuitively get back on the track toward the kind of love and support we all deserve: unconditional love and support from others that come from their knowledge of your true self. The friends I described then—Sarah, Lynne, Cheri—are still my closest friends and stood up for me at my wedding, as did my newer dear friends and supportive relatives, like my sister-in-law and cousin. And, as Merle describes, the biggest turnaround for me, because it was the one most needed and spurred from the insecurities I had surrounding my father, was my turnaround with men. As Merle already announced, the man I said those wedding vows to quite a few years ago is the charismatic actor introduced on these pages. I was fortunate to come across him after my therapy when I felt highly self-actualized, extremely self-confident, and independent, and when, most importantly, even at just twenty-two years old, I knew precisely for what I should be looking. He is an incredibly warm, loving person, who, most importantly, would never think of asking another human being to be anyone other than exactly who she is and yearns to be, and who then uniquely cherishes her for that entire spectrum of traits. That meshes completely with my own values of how I treat people, especially him, so we have had an incredibly strong, and yet infinitely flexible, unbreakable bond through the years.

Also, you might note, there's little mention in the last part of the journal of food or weight or body measurements. Once I understood the underlying reasons and the illogic associated with it, I have never been trapped or obsessed by that since. I have gained weight and lost weight—remember, that can sometimes purely be a result of taking in too few or too many calories and expending too many or too few calories—but, since those initial illuminations, none of that has ever involved self-torture or any type of obsessive or compulsive behavior, or even any guilt. I don't have to tell you how it happened. You have seen what a long, complex process was involved. And Merle has provided incredibly illuminating additional information and analysis in the most thorough and helpful mode I have ever read concerning eating disorders.

I have to say, as I sit in front of my computer that is working on a national newspaper syndicate's deadline time and a book publisher's deadline time, that my dreams really did come true. Not just career dreams or romance dreams, but the dreams of my innermost depths: I'm not imprisoned by that disease! I am free as a person and a woman. Needless to say, although there is pressure to do so in our current society, neither women nor men need to be slaves to their bodies or their scales. Just walk away and seek help! It may be a long walk, but that will only make you stronger.

Resource List

EATING DISORDER ORGANIZATIONS AND WEBSITES

If you would like to learn more about eating disorders and how to find help for you or someone you love, there are a number of eating disorder organizations and websites that can provide information free of charge. The following is a list of well-known, reliable sources of educational information. This list is by no means exhaustive—but it is an excellent place to start.

AED—Academy for Eating Disorders
www.aedweb.org
Website provides information on eating disorders and a directory of professionals in your area.

Alliance for Eating Disorders Awareness
www.eatingdisorderinfo.org
Website provides information on identification and causes of eating disorders, how to get help, and advice for parents and males.
PO Box 13155
North Palm Beach, Florida 33408-3155
866-662-1235
561-841-0900
info@eatingdisorderinfo.org

Body Positive.com
www.bodypositive.com
Website looks at ways to "feel good in the bodies we have." Provides information and resources on such topics as children and weight, size acceptance, hunger and satiety, and more.

Eating Disorder Referral and Information Center
www.edreferral.com
Provides information on eating disorders and treatment resources. Website offers comprehensive database of treatment professionals that is updated daily.

IAEDP—International Association of Eating Disorders Professionals Foundation
www.IAEDP.com
Website has a directory of treatment professionals to help you find a therapist in your area.
PO Box 1295
Pekin, Illinois 61555-1295
800-800-8126
309-346-3341
iaedpmembers@earthlink.net

ANAD—National Association of Anorexia Nervosa and Associated Disorders

www.ANAD.org

Offers hotline counseling, free support groups, referrals, and education and prevention programs. ANAD is also an advocacy organization.

PO Box 7

Highland Park, Illinois 60035

847-831-3438

anad20@aol.com

NEDIC—National Eating Disorder Information Center

www.nedic.ca

Canadian organization providing information and resources on eating disorders. Offers directory of treatment professionals in Canada.

866-NEDIC-20

416-340-4156

nedic@uhn.on.ca

NEDA—National Eating Disorders Association

www.nationaleatingdisorders.org

Offers toll-free information and referral helpline and online referrals. Provides extensive information on eating disorders and related topics. Sponsors National Eating Disorders Awareness Week.

603 Stewart Street

Suite 803

Seattle, Washington 98101

800-931-2237

info@NationalEatingDisorders.org

Something-fishy.org

www.something-fishy.org

Provides education and information to raise awareness of eating disorders, online support, and a directory of treatment options.

BOOKS ON EATING DISORDERS

We hope that reading this book has been helpful if you or someone you love might be suffering from an eating disorder. There are a number of fine books available that can provide additional insights on eating disorders. Michael Levine was instrumental in compiling this resource list. His excellent book (listed below) also contains a highly extensive list of resources.

Cash, T.F. *The Body Image Workbook: An 8 Step Program for Learning to Like Your Looks.* Oakland, CA: New Harbinger Publications, 1997.

Costin, C. *The Eating Disorder Sourcebook: A Comprehensive Guide to the Causes, Treatments, and Prevention of Eating Disorders.* McGraw-Hill, 1999.

Costin, C. *Your Dieting Daughter: Is She Dying for Attention?* New York: Brunner /Mazel, 1997.

Hall, L. *Full Lives: Women Who Have Freed Themselves From Food and Weight Obsession.* Carlsbad, CA: Gurze Books, 1993.

Kater, K. *Real Kids Come in All Sizes: 10 Essential Lessons to Build Your Child's Body Esteem.* New York: Random House, 2004.

Kelly, J. *Dads and Daughters: How to Inspire, Understand, and Support Your Daughter When She is Growing Up So Fast.* New York: Broadway Books, 2003.

Levine, M., Smolak, L. *The Prevention of Eating Problems and Eating Disorders.* Mahwah, NJ: Lawrence Erlbaum Associates, 2005. (This book contains an extensive resource list including an excellent list for educators and clinicians, minority groups, and advocacy groups.)

Maine, M. *Body Wars: Making Peace With Women's Bodies.* Carlsbad, CA: Gurze Books, 1999.

Miller, C. *My Name Is Caroline.* iUniverse, 2000.

Natenshon, A. *When Your Child Has an Eating Disorder: A Step-by-Step Workbook for Parents and Other Caregivers.* Jossey-Bass, 1999.

Siegel, M., Brisman, J., Weinshel, M. *Surviving an Eating Disorder: Strategies for Family and Friends.* New York: Harper Collins, 1997.

Zerbe, K. *The Body Betrayed: A Deeper Understanding of Women, Eating Disorders, and Treatment.* Washington, DC: American Psychiatric Press, 1993.

TREATMENT CENTERS

Finding the right center or hospital for the treatment of an eating disorder is an important task. The following treatment facilities offer a variety of outpatient, inpatient, and residential programs. All are excellent, but this is by no means an exhaustive list. If you are seeking help for yourself or for someone you care about, you should use this list as a stepping-stone to your own research. Remember to ask questions and feel comfortable and confident with your ultimate selection. Good luck!

Avalon Hills
Adolescent Treatment Facility
7852 West 600 North
Petersboro, Utah 84325
800-330-0490 or 435-753-3686
Adult Treatment Facility
8530 South 500 West
Paradise, Utah 84328
800-330-0490 or 435-245-4537
www.avalonhills.org
Avalon Hills provides a unique program where clients receive individual psychotherapy as well as a variety of group therapy and classes on topics such as nutrition, compulsion and stress manage-ment, and skills building. Avalon Hills offers animal-assisted therapy and animal activities, and the therapeutic use of outdoor experiences and challenges for discovery and growth.

Castlewood
800 Holland Road
St. Louis, Missouri 63021
888-822-8938
info@castlewoodtc.com
www.castlewoodtc.com
Castlewood offers residential treatment, partial hospitalization, day treatment, and outpatient programs for the compre-

hensive treatment of eating disorders as well as other co-existing disorders, such as trauma, attachment disorder, addictions, and more.

Center for Change

1790 N. State Street
Orem, Utah 84057
801-224-8255 or 888-224-8250
info@centerforchange.com
www.centerforchange.com

The Center provides treatment of eating disorders for teens and adults in a mountain environment, and accepts women ages 13 and older. Includes a school program for teens and family week (Thursday through Monday) monthly. The Center treats "the whole human being—spiritual, emotional, and physical," and works with the concept of intuitive eating. It offers a full continuum of inpatient, residential day and outpatient treatment.

Center for Discovery and Adolescent Change

4136 Ann Arbor Rd.
Lakewood, California 90712
800-760-3934
info@centerfordiscovery.com
www.centerfordiscovery.com

The Center is entirely devoted to treating adolescents from ages 11 to 19. It offers an intensive residential program for eating disorders and dual diagnosis, a daily school program, as well as twice-weekly individual and family group meetings. It provides continuum of care with partial hospital and day treatment programs. The Center provides a strong family-systems approach and psychoeducational component. Emphasis is on nutrition, reflective meals, and high-challenge outings.

Children's Hospital of Omaha

402-955-6190 or 800-642-8822
www.chsomaha.org

Children's Hospital and Creighton University School of Medicine offer a unique eating disorders program for children and adolescents under age 20. The program includes inpatient, day hospital, and outpatient services for youngsters with eating disorders and problems.

Comenzar de Nuevo, AC, Foundation and Eating Disorders Center

Humberto Lobo 240-8 Colonia Del Valle
Garza García
NL México 66220
52-81-8129-4683 or 52-81-8129-4684
comenzardenuevo@axtel.net
www.comenzardenuevo.org

This Mexican clinic has a twelve-bed residential treatment center with a bilingual staff. The program costs about one-third the amount of a similar program in the United States. The foundation works for the awareness, education, and prevention of eating disorders. In addition, it is a recognized leader in training professionals as well as enhancing community involvement in the field of eating disorders in Latin America as well as the United States.

CRC Health Group

408-998-7260 or 866-540-5240
www.crchealth.com

CRC sets the standards of excellence in the treatment of eating disorders and other behavioral health disorders. CRC integrates the different treatment interventions and customizes treatment to the unique needs of each person. Treatment emphasizes the physical, men-

tal, emotional and spiritual transformation of the individual. In addition to
the residential inpatient facilities located
in home-like settings, day program and
intensive outpatient treatment is offered.

Centers for the treatment of eating disorders include:

Center of Hope of the Sierras
  (Reno, NV)

Montecatini (San Diego, CA)

Life Healing Center (Santa Fe, NM)

Sierra Tucson (Tucson, AZ)

Laureate Treatment Center

6655 South Yale Avenue
Tulsa, Oklahoma 74136
918-491-3702
www.laureate.com
*This psychiatric clinic and hospital is
a part of the St. Francis Health System.
It is a full-spectrum hospital with separate programs for adolescents and adults.
Laureate has been in operation for two
decades and is considered a center of
excellence for the research and treatment
of eating disorders.*

Monte Nido

310-457-9958
www.montenido.com
*Monte Nido is a unique residential eating
disorder program developed by Carolyn
Costin. Carolyn, recovered herself, has been
treating eating disorders for 30 years. She,
and her staff, many of whom are also recovered, offer comprehensive treatment and
serve as role models that full recovery is
possible. This is individualized treatment at
its best in a natural, serene environment.
To learn more about the philosophy of
Monte Nido, you can refer to Carolyn's*

books, The Eating Disorder Sourcebook
and Your Dieting Daughter.

Renfrew Center

475 Spring Lane
Philadelphia, Pennsylvania 19128
800-Renfrew
info@renfrewcenter.com
www.renfrewcenter.com
*Renfrew Center provides treatment for
adolescents as young as 14. The
inpatient centers accept women only.
Outpatient centers accept men and
women. Programs include inpatient,
day treatment, intensive outpatient,
and outpatient individual and group
treatment. School and family treatment
is offered for teens. Inpatient centers are
located in Philadelphia, PA and Greater
Ft. Lauderdale, FL. Outpatient centers
include Bryn Mawr, PA; Wilton, CT;
New York City; Ridgewood, NJ;
Philadelphia, PA; and Coconut Creek, FL.
Renfrew has treated over 45,000 patients,
and was the first freestanding residential
center for eating disorders. Additional
treatment tracks target trauma, addictions, exercise abuse, and 30 something.
Renfrew Center Foundation is a leader in
training and education for professionals.*

Rogers Memorial Hospital

800-767-4411
www.rogershospital.org
*Eating Disorder Services provides men
and women with comprehensive, effective treatment for eating disorders. Three
levels of care are offered—inpatient,
residential, and partial hospitalization.
The multidisciplinary approach provides
individualized treatment, and the unique
residential treatment plan has a separate
program for males. To support recovery,*

services also include outpatient referrals and an alumni association. The hospital has four locations in Wisconsin, and treats ages 12 and up.

Sheppard Pratt Hospital

6535 N. Charles Street
Suite 300
Baltimore, Maryland 21204
410-938-5252 or 800-627-0330
www.sheppardpratt.org

Sheppard Pratt accepts both men and women, and provides treatment for adolescents as young as 11. The hospital offers an extremely individualized program including food plans with respect for dietary and religious needs. It offers comprehensive school and family programs. Inpatient care lasts approximately two weeks and continuity of care day treatment is about three weeks with a transition to an intensive outpatient program.

University of Iowa Hospitals and Clinics—Eating and Weight Disorder Program

319-384-8999 or 877-384-8999
www.uihealthcare.com / depts / eatingdisorders / index.html

Arnold E. Andersen, MD, is the Clinical Director of this program. Dr. Andersen has had extensive experience with males and

eating disorders. The program provides a comprehensive psychological, medical, and social approach to the treatment of eating disorders. Individualized care includes inpatient, partial hospitalization, and outpatient programs.

Westwind Eating Disorder Recovery Centre

458 14th Street
Brandon, Manitoba R7A 4T3
Canada
888-353-3372
www.westwind.mb.ca

Westwind is Canada's only private treatment facility treating anorexia, bulimia, and related eating disorders in a home-like setting. Treatment is collaborative and personal, and includes daily group and individual therapy. The affordable rate is only $300 per day.

Women's Center at Pine Grove

3875 Veteran's Memorial Drive
Hattiesburg, Mississippi 39403
888-574-HOPE
info@pinegrove-treatment.com
www.pinegrove-treatment.com

The Women's Center offers eating disorders as well as dual diagnosis treatment. It is a program "designed by women, for women addressing the needs of a woman's body, soul, and spirit."

About the Authors

Lisa Messinger earned her Bachelor of Arts degree, cum laude, in print journalism from the University of Southern California with a minor in the Study of Women and Men in Society. She has been a nationally syndicated columnist for Copley News Service for more than a decade, where she currently writes two weekly columns. She is also a longtime health, nutrition, and food newspaper editor and reporter; and since 2003, has been integral to the daily operations of various health studies for the world-renowned RAND Corporation think tank. Lisa won first place nationally for her nutrition writing from both the Association of Food Journalists and the National Council Against Health Fraud, and was named "Woman of the Year" by the University of Southern California Gender Studies department.

An award-winning public speaker, Lisa has appeared on more than seventy-five television shows and has spoken nationwide regarding eating disorders. She is also the author or co-author of seven nutrition books, including *Why Should I Eat Better? Simple Answers to All Your Nutritional Questions.*

Merle Cantor Goldberg, LCSW, DSCW, CEDS, received a diplomate in clinical social work from the University of Maryland, and has specialized in treating eating disorders for over thirty-five years. Over this period, she has served as a training leader for the International Association of Eating Disorders. Currently the Executive Director of Associates in Psychotherapy, she has appeared on many radio and television shows and is a highly sought-after lecturer. The author's articles have been published in numerous newspapers and magazines, and she is co-author of *Weight-Loss Surgery* and *The Human Circle.*

Index

12 MAGIC WANDS

The Art of Meeting Life's Challenges

G.G. Bolich, PhD

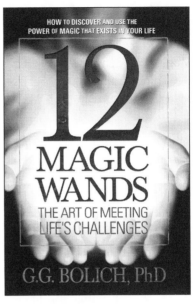

HOW TO DISCOVER AND USE THE
POWER OF MAGIC THAT EXISTS IN YOUR LIFE

12
MAGIC
WANDS
THE ART OF MEETING
LIFE'S CHALLENGES

G.G. BOLICH, PhD

Magic exists. It is everywhere. It surrounds us and infuses us. It holds the power to transform us. It isn't always easy to see, but then again, it wouldn't be magic if it was. Counselor and educator G.G. Bolich has written *Twelve Magic Wands*—a unique and insightful guide for recognizing the magic in our lives, and then using it to improve our physical, mental, and spiritual selves. It provides a step-by-step program that empowers the reader to meet and conquer life's consistent challenges.

The book begins by explaining what magic is and where it abides. It then offers twelve magic "wands" that can transform one's life for the better. Each wand provides practical tools and exercises to gain control over a specific area, such as friendship and love. Throughout the book, the author presents inspiring true stories of people who have used the magic in their lives to both help themselves and point the way to others.

The world can be a difficult place. Loneliness, disappointments, tragedies, and dead ends can sometimes seem insurmountable. Losing the magic in one's life can make it even more difficult. *Twelve Magic Wands* provides real ways to make it better—first inside, and then out.

About the Author

Dr. G.G. Bolich received his Master's of Divinity from George Fox University in Newberg, Oregon. He earned his first PhD in educational leadership from Gonzaga University in Spokane, Washington, and a second in psychology from The Union Institute in Cincinnati, Ohio. Currently a professor at Webster University in South Carolina, Dr. Bolich has taught courses at the university level since 1975. He also provides private counseling, specializing in trauma resolution, and is the published author of six titles and numerous articles in the fields of psychology, religion, and spirituality. Among his published works are *Psyche's Child, Introduction to Religion,* and *The Christian Scholar.*

$15.95 • 160 pages • 6 x 9-inch quality paperback • ISBN 0-7570-0086-X

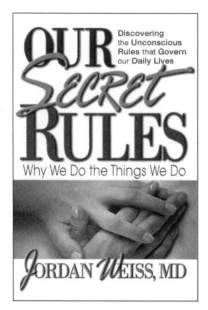

OUR SECRET RULES

Why We Do the Things We Do

Jordan Weiss, MD

We all live our lives according to a set of rules that regulate our behaviors. Some rules are quite clear. These are conscious beliefs we hold dear. Others, however, are unconscious. These are our secret rules, and when we do things that go against them, we experience stress, anxiety, apprehension, and emotional exhaustion—and we never know why. That is, until now. In *Our Secret Rules,* Dr. Jordan Weiss offers a unique system that helps uncover our most secret rules.

The book begins by explaining the important roles that conscious and unconscious rules play in our daily existence. Each chapter focuses on a key area of our lives—money, religion, gender identification, work, friendships, health, power, personal expression, marriage, and sex. Within each chapter, there are challenging questions for the reader. The answers provide a personal look at how we are likely to behave when faced with specific situations. Each chapter ends with an analysis of potential answers that is designed to reveal the extent of our secret rules.

Our Secret Rules concludes by explaining how we can use our newly gained insights to improve the way we feel about ourselves and others. For once we are aware of our rules, we can then learn to live within their boundaries, or we can attempt to change them. And as we do, we can enjoy the benefits of happier, more harmonious lives.

About the Author

Dr. Jordan Weiss received his medical degree from the University of Illinois Medical School in Chicago. With an emphasis on the body-mind-spirit connection, he has worked at several leading complementary medical centers. A practicing psychiatrist for over twenty years, Dr. Weiss currently works at Irvine's Center for Psychoenergetic Therapy in California. He is the author of several published articles on emotional responses, and is a highly regarded speaker.

$11.95 • 184 pages • 6 x 9-inch quality paperback • ISBN 0-7570-0010-X

For more information about our books, visit our website at www.squareonepublishers.com